SUMMARY OF DRUG INTERACTIONS WITH ORAL CONTRACEPTIVES

Advice for Management

A variety of drugs has been reported to reduce the efficacy of oral contraceptives (Table 1). Conversely, theoretically, combined oral contraceptives may alter the pharmacotherapeutic effect of other drugs administered concurrently. The available evidence is judged by the following qualifications in decreasing likelihood: 'established,' 'probable,' 'suspected,' possible or 'doubtful.'

Reduced Oral Contraceptive Efficacy

Table 1 Drugs reported to reduce the efficacy of oral contraceptives

Drug	Mechanism of action	Documentation level	Management
Hydantoins Barbiturates Primidone Carbamazepine	Liver enzyme induction	Established	Alternative drug (1); if this is not feasible, use a higher dose pill regimen (3)
Rifampicin	Liver enzyme induction	Established	Temporarily use extra contraceptive precautions (2) or use a higher dose pill regimen (3)
Certain antibiotics particularly penicillins and derivatives, and tetracyclines	Possibly diminished enterohepatic circulation of ethinylestradiol	Probable	Temporarily use extra contraceptive precautions (2)
Griseofulvin	Liver enzyme induction	Suspected	Temporarily use extra contraceptive precautions (2)
Other drugs (4)	Not established	Doubtful	Not applicable

(1) An alternative drug without enzyme-inducing properties should be used.

(2) In the case of short-term concurrent drug treatment, a barrier method should be used both during concurrent drug treatment and for 7 days after discontinuation. If this would continue into the next oral contraceptive tablet-free interval, the woman should skip the tablet-free interval and start the next pack as soon as she has finished the pack in use.

(3) In the case of long-term concurrent enzyme-inducing drug treatment:

 – It is recommended to prescribe as a standard starting routine a monophasic 50 µg ethinylestradiol oral contraceptive (do not prescribe an oral contraceptive with placebo tablets, every-day pill). For example, the dosage regimen with this oral contraceptive could be four packs in a row followed by a tablet-free interval of 5 or 6 days. The contraceptive efficacy of the regimen can be judged on the basis of the occurrence of irregular bleeding (IB). IB is normally reviewed during the first follow-up visit (i.e. after the first four packs have been used). However, the woman should be advised that if IB is heavy and prolonged she should return sooner.

 – If IB is too frequent:

 ● Increase the ethinylestradiol dose either by prescribing a regimen of two sub-50 µg ethinylestradiol oral contraceptive tablets/day (i.e. two tablets with 30–35 µg ethinylestradiol/tablet) or a regimen of one 50 µg ethinylestradiol oral contraceptive tablet + one sub-50 µg ethinylestradiol oral contraceptive tablet/day.

 ● If IB still continues, increase the ethinylestradiol dose further to two 50 µg ethinylestradiol oral contraceptive tablets/day.

 ● If the above options are still not successful in controlling IB, use of an alternative contraceptive method should be advised.

Note that after enzyme-inducing medication has been stopped, liver enzyme induction may be sustained during a period of about 4 weeks. Therefore, during this period, it is necessary either to stay on the higher dose oral contraceptive regimen or, when the woman resumes low-dose oral contraceptive use, in addition, to use a barrier method.

(4) A number of other drugs have been suggested to cause oral contraceptive failure. The following drugs have been mentioned in the literature: acetyl salicylic acid (aspirin), activated charcoal (and other adsorbents), aminopyrine, antidepressants (tricyclic), antipyrine, ascorbic acid, chloramphenicol, chlorcyclizine, chlordiazepoxide, chloroquine, chlorpromazine, cholestyramine, cimetidine, clindamycin, co-trimoxazole, dapsone, diazepam, diazoxide, dichloralphenazone, dihydroergotamine, erythromycin, ethosuximide, glutethimide, ibuprofen, indomethacin, isoniazid, laxatives, meprobamate, neomycin, nitrofurantoin, paracetamol (acetaminophen), phenacetin, phenylbutazone, phenylephedrine, promethazine, sulfonamides, thyroid hormone.

Influence of Oral Contraceptives on the Pharmacotherapeutic Effect of Other Drugs

Occasionally, reports have appeared, suggesting that the use of oral contraceptives may influence the pharmacotherapeutic effect of other drugs. These include: analgesics, antidepressants, antimalarial drugs, benzodiazepines, β-blockers, corticosteroids, hypoglycaemic drugs, oral anticoagulants and theophylline. The documentation level regarding these interactions varies from 'possible' to 'probable'. However, so far no evidence has been obtained indicating that clinically significant effects occur that would require adjustment of the dose or prescription of an alternative medication.

From Geurts, T.B.P., Goorissen, E.M. and Sitsen, J.M.A. (1993)
Summary of Drug Interactions with Oral Contraceptives
(Carnforth: Parthenon Publishing)

SUMMARY
OF DRUG
INTERACTIONS
WITH ORAL
CONTRACEPTIVES

T.B.P. GEURTS,
E.M. GOORISSEN AND J.M.A. SITSEN

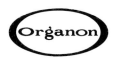

The Parthenon Publishing Group
International Publishers in Medicine, Science & Technology

Casterton Hall, Carnforth,
Lancs LA6 2LA, UK

One Blue Hill Plaza, Pearl River,
New York 10965, USA

Published in the UK by
The Parthenon Publishing Group Ltd.
Casterton Hall
Carnforth, Lancs LA6 2LA, England

Published in North America by
The Parthenon Publishing Group Inc.
One Blue Hill Plaza
PO Box 1564, Pearl River
New York 10965, USA

Copyright © 1993 Organon International bv

British Library Cataloguing in Publication Data
Geurts, T.B.P.
 Summary of Drug Interactions with Oral Contraceptives
 I. Title
 615

 ISBN: 1-85070-518-6

Library of Congress Cataloging-in-Publication Data
Geurts, T.B.P.
 Summary of drug interactions with oral contraceptives / T.B.P.
Geurts, E.M. Goorissen, and J.M.A. Sitsen.
  p. cm
 Includes bibliographical references and index.
 ISBN 1-85070-518-6
 1. Oral contraceptives--Physiological effect. 2. Drug
interactions. I. Goorissen, E.M. II. Sitsen, J.M.A.
III. Title. IV. Title: Drug interactions with oral contraceptives.
 [DNLM: 1. Drug Interactions. 2. Contraceptives, Oral. OV 177
G396s 1993]
RG137.5.G48 1993
615'. 766--dc20
DNLM/DLC
for Library of Congress   93-25435
                                                                CIP

The authors, reviewers and editors of the book have made every effort to present
an accurate overview of facts known and views expressed in the literature thus far
(i.e. November, 1992).

However, new facts may become known and further opinions may be expressed.
Also, no compilation of published information can be entirely objective, complete
and free from human error.

Therefore, the reader must use his or her own judgement when referring to this
publication and consult other sources of information if necessary, in addition to
the product information supplied by the manufacturer of any drug to be administered or prescribed.

Typeset by Rowland & Hird, Lancaster, Lancs
Printed and bound in Great Britain by Butler & Tanner Ltd.,
Frome and London

Contents

Introduction

When prescribing drugs the physician has to take into consideration that concurrent administration may lead to drug interactions, i.e. the alteration of the effects of one drug by the effects of another drug. This is particularly important in the case of oral contraceptives, which are agents usually taken continuously for many years.

Interactions due to the concurrent administration of an oral contraceptive and another drug may have two different implications: either altered efficacy of the pill (which may lead to unintended pregnancy), or an altered pharmacological effect of the other drug (and, occasionally, as a result of the latter, even the occurrence of adverse effects).

The first report on loss of contraceptive efficacy appeared in 1971 by Reimers and Jezek who observed an increased incidence of intermenstrual bleeding in oral contraceptive users receiving rifampicin and other antituberculous drugs. This observation was followed by numerous other case reports and experimental studies specifically investigating the mechanisms of interaction. The possibility that drug interactions could jeopardize oral contraceptive efficacy is still gaining importance, because over the years, steroid dosage with the pill has been reduced substantially and this trend is still continuing. It should be obvious that impairment of contraceptive activity bears clinical significance, since the ultimate result may be accidental pregnancy. On the other hand, the arguments raised to date with regard to the clinical consequences of pill-induced alterations of the pharmacological effects of other drugs are, generally speaking, not very strong.

In this volume, both types of interactions will be reviewed, paying particular attention to the underlying mechanisms of interaction.

When judging the clinical impact of drug interactions, it is crucial to use strict definitions. This is particularly true in view of the fact that, although in total the available documentation is extensive, it often concerns fragmentary data or contradictory findings. Looking for proper criteria and definitions for classifying clinical significance (determined by documentation level and severity) in major handbooks on drug interactions, the authors decided to adopt the classification system as used by *Drug Interaction Facts* (DIF, 1993, updated quarterly).

Indicating the clinical significance of reported interactions with oral contraceptives, they have consistently applied the criteria as provided by DIF. In addition, and whenever relevant, recommendations will be given for the management of oral contraceptive users who need multidrug treatment.

Chapter 1:
Mechanisms of Drug Interactions

1.1 INTRODUCTION

Drug interactions may result from changes in either the pharmacokinetics or the pharmacodynamics of the drugs involved (Brodie and Feely, 1988). Consequently, this classification will be used in the following general information on the mechanisms of drug interactions (Sections 1.2 and 1.3, respectively).

1.2 PHARMACOKINETIC INTERACTIONS

Pharmacokinetic interactions may take place at any stage of absorption, distribution, metabolism or excretion. With oral contraceptives, there is evidence of substantial differences in the pharmacokinetics of both ethinylestradiol and the progestagen component within and between populations (Back and Orme, 1984). Consequently, the chance of drug interaction occurring will, to a large extent, depend on how contraceptive steroids are metabolized in a given individual.

1.2.1 REDUCED ABSORPTION OR REABSORPTION

A drug may influence both the rate and the extent of absorption of another drug by the following mechanisms:

(1) By decreasing its solubility in water;

(2) By adsorption onto insoluble materials;

(3) By alteration of gastrointestinal pH; and

(4) By causing increased or decreased gastrointestinal motility (Griffin, 1981).

In theory, the absorption of oral contraceptives may be affected by any one of these mechanisms.

A change in the rate of absorption of a drug with a long elimination half-life would probably have a small clinical effect if its total absorption were not altered. However, if a drug has a short elimination half-life or if a rapid effect is needed, a delayed absorption can be clinically significant. Interactions decreasing the extent of drug absorption are especially likely to be significant if the affected drug (or 'object drug' (Grahame-Smith and Aronson, 1992)) has a narrow therapeutic range, such as current low-dose oral contraceptives.

The increased gastrointestinal motility (leading to diarrhea) secondary to alteration of gut bacterial flora, which may be caused by penicillins and certain other antibiotics, could also be a potential offender of oral contraceptive efficacy. In addition, gastroenteritis has long been considered as being a potential cause of malabsorption of contraceptive steroids (Brodie and Feely, 1988; Kerremans, 1989).

Further, drug interaction-induced changes in gut wall metabolism (due to increased cytochrome P_{450} activity or competition for conjugation mechanisms) have been recognized as being a possible cause of an alteration in the bioavailability of estrogens. The bioavailability of progestagens, however, remains unaffected (Back *et al.*, 1980a;1981a; Griffin, 1981; Back *et al.*, 1981b).

Reduced reabsorption of contraceptive steroids from the gut could be another cause of contraceptive failure. Contraceptive steroids are metabolized in the liver to form inactive conjugates. Ethinylestradiol, for example, is well absorbed from the gut, but, on average, 60% of the dose is metabolized on its first-pass in the body to form sulfate and glucuronide conjugates. Sulfation occurs primarily in the small intestinal mucosa (Back *et al.*, 1981a; 1982; Rogers *et al.*, 1987), while conjugation with glucuronic acid occurs mainly in the liver (Helton *et al.*, 1976; Sahlberg *et al.*, 1981). These conjugates are excreted in the bile and are partly broken down by hydrolytic enzymes produced by gut bacteria to release free and active steroids that are then reabsorbed. This cycle of events is called the enterohepatic circulation.

This enterohepatic circulation would be interrupted if, for example, antibiotics were to inhibit gut bacteria. The microflora of the gastrointestinal tract in man responsible for the deconjugation of ethinylestradiol include mainly obligate anaerobic bacteria such as clostridia, *Bacteroides* spp., lactose-fermenting coliform bacteria and some staphylococci (Chapman, 1981).

Antibiotics may kill the clostridia responsible for the hydrolytic process. This may lead to loss of conjugates (which are too hydrophilic to be absorbed), thus diminishing the overall bioavailability of ethinylestradiol to a possibly ineffective contraceptive level. However, although ethinylestradiol undergoes this enterohepatic circulation in women to a variable extent, animal studies have shown that progestagens do so only as reduced and therefore inactive metabolites (Back *et al.*, 1978; Adlercreutz *et al.*, 1984). Furthermore, although the bacteria in the gut possess enzymes that hydrolyze glucuronide conjugates, there is no clear evidence that they can also deal with sulfate conjugates (D'Arcy, 1986; Shenfield, 1986; Brodie and Feely, 1988).

1.2.2 ENZYME INDUCTION

Enzyme induction is the stimulation of the production of enzymes involved in the metabolism of drugs. The latter takes place via binding of the drug to intracellular receptors mainly in the liver (but also in other tissues such as the intestine) resulting in increased enzyme synthesis and increased enzymatic activity. This drug-metabolizing enzyme system has two major functions: first, rapid breakdown of a variety of endogenous and exogenous substances into inactive metabolites; and second, transformation of these substances from lipid-soluble into water-soluble compounds which can then be excreted via the urine and/or feces. Drug metabolism reactions consist of Phase I biotransformations, such as oxidation, reduction and hydrolysis, and Phase II biotransformations, which involve conjugation of the drug (or metabolite) with a small endogenous molecule.

Some environmental chemicals such as dichlorodiphenyltrichloroethane (DDT), polychlorinated biphenyls (PCBs) and hexachlorocyclohexane are metabolized very slowly by this enzyme system, which explains the accumulation of these substances (Greim, 1980).

As protein synthesis is required for enzyme induction, the maximum effect is not seen for 2–3 weeks. Enzyme induction results in accelerated metabolism of the drugs involved, with a reduction in their circulating concentration and an attenuation of their pharmacological effects. Quantitatively, the most important enzymes are the hepatic cytochrome P_{450} mixed-function oxidases which, by simply 'inserting' oxygen into drug molecules, are able to bring about numerous biotransformations, including aliphatic and aromatic hydroxylation, N-, S- and O-demethylation, deamination, dechlorination and desulfurization. These enzymes are localized principally in the microsomes, but also in other parts of the cell. The microsomal enzyme hydroxylation systems are unique in that they can be induced to some extent by a wide range of biologically and chemically unrelated compounds, including exogenous drugs, endogenous steroids and other hormones, xenobiotics, nutrients and environmental pollutants (Greim, 1980; Park and Breckenridge, 1981).

Although a wide range of agents are able to increase the activities of drug-metabolizing enzymes in animal models, the number of drugs with important enzyme-inducing properties in man is small. Therefore, it must be emphasized that only certain anticonvulsants (barbiturates, carbamazepine and phenytoin) and the antimicrobial drug, rifampicin, have appeared to be clinically important enzyme-inducing agents in man (Breckenridge, 1987).

It also appears that enzyme inducers do have several features in common, such as lipophilicity, the ability to bind to cytochrome P_{450} enzymes, and relatively long biological half-lives. However, this is not a prerequisite, since many drugs that have these properties do not induce enzyme synthesis. It is also important to note that many chemicals encountered in the environment, such as pesticides and PCBs, charcoal-broiled food (which also may contain PCBs due to the broiling process), cabbage and Brussels sprouts can also stimulate drug metabolism (Conney et al., 1976; Kappas et al., 1978; Pantuck et al., 1979).

Recently, progress has been made in unravelling the cellular basis of drug interactions with oral contraceptives in which enzyme induction is involved. This bears particular significance for ethinylestradiol. The major pathway of ethinylestradiol metabolism is 2-hydroxylation by cytochrome P_{450}. It has been argued that the specific isoenzyme responsible for estrogen 2-hydroxylation is $P_{450}IIIA4$ (previously called P_{450Nf}, but the recommended nomenclature according to Nebert et al. (1989) will be used in this review), which is a member of the $P_{450}IIIA$ subfamily (Guengerich et al., 1986; Guengerich, 1988).

Although purified $P_{450}IIIA4$ has relatively low catalytic ethinylestradiol 2-hydroxylase activity, antibodies raised to $P_{450}IIIA4$ inhibit specifically >90% of the activity in human liver microsomes. Consequently, the working hypothesis has to be that, for instance, phenobarbital and other anticonvulsant drugs induce this isoenzyme and consequently increase the rate and extent of ethinylestradiol 2-hydroxylation (Guengerich, 1988). The findings of Guengerich are supported by the data of Ball et al. (1990), who also identified the cytochrome $P_{450}IIIA$ and $P_{450}IIC$ gene subfamilies as the major ethinylestradiol-metabolizing enzyme systems, whereas they also found that these enzyme systems were inducible by both phenobarbital and phenytoin. On the other hand, these authors also found that estradiol is metabolized by enzymes from the $P_{450}IA$ (inducible by polycyclic aromatic hydrocarbon), $P_{450}IIC$ and $P_{450}IIE$

subfamilies and not by cytochrome P_{450}IIIA. From the study by Ball *et al.* (1990) it would be expected that plasma estradiol levels would be affected by smoking whereas ethinylestradiol levels would remain unaffected, which indeed is what has been found in pharmacokinetic studies (Crawford *et al.*, 1981; Jensen and Christiansen, 1988; Michnovicz *et al.*, 1988). The marked differences in selectivity of cytochrome P_{450} in estradiol and ethinylestradiol 2-hydroxylation are attributable to the D-ring 17α-substituent. Therefore, the steroid D-ring must play a role in substrate recognition for cytochrome P_{450}(Ball *et al.*, 1990).

Data on the metabolism of synthetic progestagens are not available, but there are indications that also endogenous progesterone is metabolized by cytochrome P_{450}IIIA (Batt *et al.*, 1992). This may also render synthetic progestagenic steroids susceptible for enzyme induction.

1.2.3 ENZYME INHIBITION

Most inhibitory interactions take place through the effects on hepatic enzymes. Many compounds have the potential for interfering with the metabolism of other drugs, usually by competing for binding sites on the appropriate enzymes. Other possible mechanisms are:

(1) By preventing the entrance of substrates into the cell through alteration of membrane permeability or depression of transport systems;

(2) By interfering with the degradative reactions in which the substrates are oxidatively broken down;

(3) By hindering the formation of high-energy phosphates;

(4) By hampering the biosynthesis of cytoplasmatic components;

(5) By preventing the utilization of the high-energy substances by these synthetic processes; and

(6) By affecting the reactions involved in the utilization of energy.

Most compounds that inhibit drug metabolism are assumed to act by direct inhibition of the enzyme system. The cellular basis for direct enzyme inhibition is in the cytochrome P_{450} systems and is, therefore, related to that of enzyme induction (described in Section 1.2.2).

There is evidence from animal studies that sex steroids *in vitro* inhibit competitively microsomal enzymes (Juchau and Fouts, 1966; Tephly and Mannering, 1968), but the concentrations resulting in inhibition were often supraphysiological: high-dose ethinylestradiol over 5 days has been shown to decrease cytochrome P_{450} activity in livers of male rats, and was associated with decreased turnover of the P_{450} pool (Mackinnon *et al.*, 1977).

A study in women by Chambers *et al.* (1982) suggested that the estrogenic component of oral contraceptives is responsible for inhibition of drug oxidation: women receiving a progestagen-only preparation had normal antipyrine clearance, whereas those receiving a combined oral contraceptive had impaired antipyrine elimination. However, studies in the rat have shown that cytochrome P_{450} can be also inhibited in a time- and dose-dependent way by progestagenic compounds (White and Muller-Eberhard, 1977; Ortiz de Montellano *et al.*, 1979; Ortiz de Montellano and Kunze, 1980; Blakey and White, 1986).

Inhibition is dependent on the plasma concentration of the inhibitor and may be initiated as soon as adequate plasma levels of the inhibiting drugs are attained. Drugs that inhibit cytochrome P_{450} activity include certain antibiotics such as cotrimoxazole, warfarin, monoamine oxidase inhibitors and cimetidine. When an inhibitor is withdrawn, the circulating concentration of the affected drug will decrease as a result of restored metabolic activity, with a potential loss of therapeutic efficacy. Though less predictable than induction interactions, problems with metabolic inhibition should be recognized and appropriate action taken (D'Arcy, 1986; Brodie and Feely, 1988). An example of an oral contraceptive-induced enzyme inhibitory action on the metabolism of the concurrently administered drug is the enhanced plasma concentrations of oxidatively metabolized benzodiazepines reported in oral contraceptive users. In addition, the reverse has also been reported from *in vitro* studies in human liver homogenate, i.e. certain progestagens could reduce the 2-hydroxylation of ethinylestradiol and other microsomal oxidative metabolic steps by inhibiting cytochrome P_{450}IIIA4 activity, and thus potentiate specific (hormonal) actions (Back *et al.*, 1990; Guengerich, 1990; Pazzucconi *et al.*, 1990). The effects of such interactions would not result in terms of contraceptive failure, but may appear in certain predisposed women as secondary and undesirable pharmacological actions of contraceptive preparations with enzyme inhibitory properties, e.g. increased risk of thromboembolic disorders, hypertension or diabetogenic effects.

In addition, the concurrent use of oral contraceptives with triacetyloleandomycin (an antimicrobial agent with hepatotoxic effects) has been reported to inhibit the metabolism of ethinylestradiol, leading to accumulation in the liver and has led consequently to increased hepatoxicity (D'Arcy, 1986; Kerremans, 1989; Back and Orme, 1990).

Theoretically, a number of drugs with potent enzyme inhibitory properties might delay the metabolic degradation of contraceptive steroids and/or enhance their side-effects (D'Arcy, 1986). However, the clinical relevance should not be overestimated. At an Expert Committee Meeting in April, 1991 in Washington DC, it was concluded that changes in clearance of at least 40% were considered clinically relevant for drugs with a narrow therapeutic window (e.g. theophylline); for drugs with wide therapeutic windows, even larger changes in clearance may be considered as not clinically relevant (Schentag, 1993).

1.2.4 PLASMA CARRIER PROTEIN BINDING

Plasma sex hormone binding globulin (SHBG) levels are elevated in oral contraceptive users due to an estrogen-induced synthesis of this carrier protein in the liver. SHBG binds progestagens (but not ethinylestradiol) with high affinity, to a varying degree, depending on their androgenic activity. It has been shown that SHBG binding capacity is significantly increased in women taking enzyme-inducing drugs such as certain anticonvulsants and rifampicin (Victor *et al.*, 1977; Back *et al.*, 1980b). This would lead to a decrease in the free (non-protein-bound) concentration of progestagens in plasma and could be a supportive cause of oral contraceptive failure. However, evidence supporting the fact that a reduction in the free plasma steroid concentration leads to reduced contraceptive efficacy is lacking.

A similar mechanism of action (but now with an effect on the plasma levels of a drug used concurrently with oral contraceptives) has been postulated for the interaction between oral contraceptives and corticosteroids, the latter being bound with high affinity by corticosteroid binding globulin (CBG). In oral contraceptive users, also CBG plasma levels are elevated under the influence of the estrogen component. Since it is the unbound or free corticosteroid which is biologically active, the effects of oral contraceptives on the time course of free corticosteroid levels are of pharmacological interest. The consequence of the high CBG levels is an increased protein binding of corticosteroids and thus a retarded elimination of these hormones, which in time may lead to an increased corticosteroid effect (Gustavson and Benet, 1985). On the other hand, as a result of the increased binding to CBG, a reduction in the free plasma levels of corticosteroids could also be expected, thus leading to reduced pharmacological activity. However, the clinical significance of this reported interaction remains to be elucidated. Similarly, this mechanism of action has also been postulated with regard to a possible interaction between oral contraceptives and thyroxin. Thyroxin is bound by thyroxin binding globulin (TBG), the plasma concentration of which is also elevated by the estrogen component of oral contraceptives (D'Arcy, 1986; Brodie and Feely, 1988).

1.3 PHARMACODYNAMIC INTERACTIONS

Pharmacodynamic drug interactions can be defined as the direct influence of a certain drug upon the molecular, cellular or physiological action of another drug (Verspohl, 1980). These interactions are less readily classified and identified than those affecting drug concentrations, but they are, in general, more predictable from the pharmacological actions of the drugs involved. With this type of interaction, it is possible that several different overlapping mechanisms may operate: an interaction-induced increased pharmacological effect may be accompanied by an increased incidence of adverse events. The following mechanisms have been identified:

1.3.1 SYNERGISM

1.3.1.1 Enhanced physiological effect

The most common type of interaction, in general, is a similar physiological effect (synergism) of two drugs acting on the same system, organ, cell or enzyme. For example, all drugs which have a depressant action on the central nervous system (e.g. ethanol, antihistamines, benzodiazepines) may enhance each other's sedative effects. Synergism can be divided into competitive synergism (both drugs acting via the same receptor) and functional synergism (via different sites of action).

In theory, a similar interaction could occur between an oral contraceptive (which may increase certain clotting factors) and the antifibrinolytic drug, aminocaproic acid. These two drugs would then act synergistically and thus theoretically increase the plasma concentration of certain clotting factors (D'Arcy, 1986; Brodie and Feely, 1988).

1.3.1.2 Enhanced adverse events

Occasionally, a drug interaction may lead to an increased incidence of adverse events known to occur with a particular drug (also via competitive or functional synergism). For example, the concurrent administration of aminoglycosides and cephalosporins or diuretics results in an increased incidence of oto- and nephro-toxicity (Brodie and Feely, 1988).

1.3.2 ANTAGONISM

1.3.2.1 Decreased physiological effect

In clinical practice, it is possible for interactions to result in a decreased physiological effect (antagonism). This antagonism can be divided into competitive antagonism (both drugs acting via the same receptor) and functional antagonism (via different sites of action). Some reactions are obvious, for example, β-agonists and β-antagonists (β-blockers) or vitamin K and warfarin.

The same mechanism has been suggested for possible oral contraceptive-anticoagulant interactions. Women taking combined oral contraceptives may have increased plasma concentrations of certain vitamin K-dependent clotting factors, as well as factors involved in fibrinolysis. Since oral anticoagulants act by inhibiting the synthesis of vitamin K-dependent clotting factors, it is not surprising that oral contraceptives have been reported to affect the efficacy of anticoagulants (Brodie and Feely, 1988).

1.3.2.2 Decreased adverse effect

With this type of drug interaction, usually two different physiological pathways are active concomitantly (functional antagonism). The concurrent use of antacids and non-steroidal anti-inflammatory drugs (NSAIDS) has been reported to decrease the incidence of peptic ulcer, an adverse event known to be associated with prolonged NSAID treatment (Kerremans, 1989).

Finally, an invaluable clinical application of this type of drug interaction is in the treatment of poisoning: activated charcoal is used in the acute poisoning due to, for example, salicylates or barbiturates, whereas naloxone is used to antagonize opioid-induced respiratory depression (D'Arcy, 1986; Brodie and Feely, 1988).

1.3.3 OTHER MECHANISMS

Finally, other pharmacodynamic drug interactions (which occur less frequently and bear no relevance for the purpose of this review) act via mechanisms such as indirect receptor effects, effects on cellular transport systems (synaptic blockade) and via disturbances of fluid and electrolyte balance (Brodie and Feely, 1988).

References

Adlercreutz H, Pulkkinen MO, Hämäläinen EK, Korpela JT. Studies on the role of intestinal bacteria in metabolism of synthetic and natural steroid hormones. *J Steroid Biochem* 1984;20:217–29

Back DJ, Breckenridge AM, Challiner M, *et al*. The effect of antibiotics on the enterohepatic circulation of ethinylestradiol and norethisterone in the rat. *J Steroid Biochem* 1978;9:527–31

Back DJ, Breckenridge AM, Crawford FE, *et al*. Phenobarbitone interaction with oral contraceptive steroids in the rabbit and rat. *Br J Pharmacol* 1980a;69:441–52

Back DJ, Breckenridge AM, Crawford FE, *et al*. The effect of oral contraceptive steroids and enzyme inducing drugs on sex hormone binding globulin capacity in women. *Br J Clin Pharmacol* 1980b;9:115

Back DJ, Bates M, Breckenridge AM, *et al*. The *in vitro* metabolism of ethinylestradiol, mestranol and levonorgestrel by human jejunal mucosa. *Br J Clin Pharmacol* 1981a; 11:275–8

Back DJ, Breckenridge AM, MacIver M, Orme, ML'E, Purba H, Rowe PH. Interaction of ethinylestradiol with ascorbic acid in man. *Br Med J* 1981b;282:516

Back DJ, Breckenridge AM, MacIver M, *et al*. The gut wall metabolism of ethinylestradiol and its contribution to the pre-systemic metabolism of ethinylestradiol in humans. *Br J Clin Pharmacol* 1982;13:325–30

Back DJ, MacNee CM, Orme ML'E, *et al*. An investigation of the effects of phenobarbitone on the pharmacokinetics of norethindrone in the rat using liver perfusion and everted gut sacs. *Biochem Pharmacol* 1984;33:1595–600

Back DJ, Orme ML'E. Interindividual variability in oral contraceptive disposition. *Trends Pharmacol Sci* 1984;5:480–3

Back DJ, Orme ML'E. Pharmacokinetic drug interactions with oral contraceptives. *Clin Pharmacokinet* 1990;18:472–84

References

Back DJ, Houlgrave R, Tjia JF, Ward S, Orme ML'E. Effect of the progestogens, gestodene, 3-ketodesogestrel, levonorgestrel, norethisterone and norgestimate on the oxidation of ethinylestradiol and other substrates by human liver microsomes. *J Steroid Biochem Mol Biol* 1991; 38:219–25

Ball SE, Forrester LM, Wolf CR, Back DJ. Differences in the cytochrome P_{450} isozymes involved in the 2-hydroxylation of estradiol and 17α-ethinylestradiol: relative activities of rat and human liver enzymes. *Biochem J* 1990;267:221–6

Batt AM, Siest G, Magdalou J, Gatteau MM. Enzyme induction by drugs and toxins. *Clin Chim Acta* 1992;209:109–21

Blakey DC, White INH. Destruction of cytochrome P_{450} and formation of green pigments by contraceptive steroids in rat hepatocyte suspensions. *Biochem Pharmacol* 1986;35:1561–7

Breckenridge AM. Enzyme induction in humans. Clinical aspects – an overview. *Pharmacol Ther* 1987;33:95–9

Brodie MJ, Feely J. Adverse drug interactions. *Br Med J* 1988;296:845–9

Chambers DM, Jefferson GC, Chambers M, Loudon NB. Antipyrine elimination in saliva after low-dose combined or progestogen-only contraceptive steroids. *Br J Clin Pharmacol* 1982;13:229–32

Chapman CR. Absorption and metabolism of steroid pro-drugs. *Thesis, University of Liverpool*, Liverpool 1981

Conney AH, Pantuck EJ, Hsiao KC, Garland WA, Anderson KE, Alvares AP, Kappas A. Enhanced phenacetin metabolism in human subjects fed charcoal-broiled beef. *Clin Pharmacol Ther* 1976;20:633–42

Crawford F, Back DJ, Orme ML, Breckenridge AM. Oral contraceptive plasma concentrations in smokers and non-smokers. *Br Med J* 1981;282:1829–30

D'Arcy PF. Drug interactions with oral contraceptives. *Drug Intell Clin Pharm* 1986;20:353–62

References

Grahame-Smith DG, Aronson JK. *Oxford Textbook of Clinical Pharmacology and Drug Therapy*, 2nd edn. Oxford, New York, Tokyo: Oxford University Press, 1992

Greim H. Enzyminduktion in der Leber verändert Arzneimittelwirkung. *Ned Klin* 1980;75:709–12

Griffin JP. Drug interactions occurring during absorption from the gastrointestinal tract. *Pharmacol Ther* 1981;15:79–88

Guengerich FP, Martin MV, Beaune PH, Kremers P, Wolff T, Waxman DJ. Characterization of rat and human liver microsomal cytochrome P_{450} forms involved in nifedipine oxidation, a prototype for genetic polymorphism in oxidative drug metabolism. *J Biol Chem* 1986;261:5051–60

Guengerich FP. Oxidation of 17α-ethinylestradiol by human liver cytochrome P_{450}. *Mol Pharmacol* 1988;33:500–8

Guengerich FP. Mechanism-based inactivation of human liver microsomal cytochrome P_{450}IIIA4 by gestodene. *Chem Res Toxicol* 1990;3:363–71

Gustavson LE, Benet LZ. The macromolecular binding of prednisone in plasma of healthy volunteers including pregnant women and oral contraceptive users. *J Pharmacokinet Biopharm* 1985;13:561–9

Helton ED, Williams MC, Goldzieher JW. Human urinary and liver conjugates of 17α-ethinylestradiol. *Steroids* 1976;27:851–67

Jensen J, Christiansen C. Effect of smoking on serum lipoproteins and bone mineral content during postmenopausal hormone replacement therapy. *Am J Obstet Gynecol* 1988;159:820–5

Juchau MR, Fouts JR. Effects of norethynodrel and progesterone on hepatic microsomal drug-metabolizing enzyme systems. *Biochem Pharmacol* 1966;15:891–8

Kerremans ALM. Klinisch belangrijke geneesmiddeleninteracties. *Ned Tijdschr Geneeskd* 1989; 133:148–51

Kappas A, Alvares AP, Anderson KE, Pantuck EJ, Chang R, Conney AH. Effect of charcoal-broiled beef on antipyrine and theophylline metabolism. *Clin Pharmacol Ther* 1978;23:445–50

References

Mackinnon M, Sutherland E, Simon FE. Effects of ethinyl-estradiol on hepatic microsomal proteins and the turnover of cytochrome P_{450}. *J Lab Clin Med* 1977;90:1096–106

Michnovicz JJ, Naganuma H, Hershkopf RJ, Bradlow HL, Fishman J. Increased urinary catechol estrogen excretion in female smokers. *Steroids* 1988;52:69–83

Nebert DW, Nelson DR, Adesnik M, Coon MJ, Estabrook RW, Gonzalez FJ, *et al.* The P_{450} superfamily: updated listing of all genes and recommended nomenclature for the chromosomal loci. *DNA* 1989;8:1–13

Ortiz de Montellano PR, Kunze KL, Yost GS, Mico BA. Self-catalyzed destruction of cytochrome P_{450}: covalent binding of ethinyl sterols to prosthetic heme. *Proc Natl Acad Sci USA* 1979;76:746–9

Ortiz de Montellano PR, Kunze KL. Self-catalyzed inactivation of hepatic cytochrome P_{450} by ethinyl substrates. *J Biol Chem* 1980;255:5578–85

Pantuck EJ, Pantuck CB, Garland WA, *et al.* Stimulatory effect of Brussels sprouts and cabbage on human drug metabolism. *Clin Pharmacol Ther* 1979;25:88–95

Park BK, Breckenridge AM. Clinical implications of enzyme induction and enzyme inhibition. *Clin Pharmacokinet* 1981;6:1–24

Pazzucconi F, Calabresi L, Franceschini G, *et al.* Both gestodene and desogestrel-containing oral contraceptives reduce antipyrine clearance by impairing microsomal oxidative metabolism. *Eur J Pharmacol* 1990;183:1758

Reimers D, Jezek A. The simultaneous use of rifampicin and other tuberculosis agents with oral contraceptives. *Prax Pneumol* 1971; 25:255–62

Rogers SM, Back DJ, Orme ML'E. Intestinal metabolism of ethinylestradiol and paracetamol *in vitro*: studies using Ussing Chambers. *Br J Clin Pharmacol* 1987;23:727–34

Sahlberg B-L, Axelson M, Collins DJ, Sjovall J. Analysis of isomeric ethinylestradiol glucuronides in urine. *J Chromatography* 1981;217:453–61

References

Schentag JJ. Assessment of pharmacokinetic drug interactions in clinical drug development. In: Yacobi A, Skelly JP, Shah VP, Benet LZ, eds. *Integration of Pharmacokinectics, Pharmacodynamics and Toxicokinetics in Rational Drug Development*. New York: Plenum Press, 1993: 149–57

Shenfield GM. Drug interactions with oral contraceptive preparations. *Med J Aust* 1986;144:205–11

Tephly TR, Mannering GJ. Inhibition of drug metabolism. V. Inhibition of drug metabolism by steroids. *Mol Pharmacol* 1968;4:10–14

Verspohl EJ. Pharmakodynamische Wechselwirkungen zwischen Arzneistoffen. *Med Monatsschr Pharm* 1980;3:228–40

Victor A, Lundberg PO, Johansson EDB. Induction of sex hormone binding globulin by phenytoin. *Br Med J* 1977;2:934–5

White INH, Muller-Eberhard U. Decreased liver cytochrome P_{450} in rats caused by norethindrone or ethinylestradiol. *Biochem J* 1977;166:57–64

Chapter 2:
Criteria for Assessment of Clinical Significance

2.1 INTRODUCTION

In order to decide whether reports of drug–oral contraceptive interactions would require specific management decisions, one has to indicate their clinical significance. After reviewing the set-up and the various conclusions arrived at by major handbooks on drug interactions, preference has been given to the adoption of criteria for classification offered by *Drug Interaction Facts* (DIF, St. Louis, JB Lippincott Co.).

2.2 CLINICAL SIGNIFICANCE

When evaluating any potential drug interaction, a primary concern is the clinical relevance or significance of the interaction. Significance relates to the type and magnitude of the effect and, subsequently, to the necessity of monitoring the patient or altering therapy to avoid potentially adverse consequences. Clinical significance is determined by the combination of severity and documentation level of the interaction concerned.

2.2.1 SEVERITY

The potential severity of the interaction is particularly important in assessing the risk versus benefit of therapeutic alternatives. With appropriate dosage adjustments or modification of the administration schedule, the negative effects of most interactions can be avoided. Three degrees of severity are defined:

Major: The effects are potentially life-threatening or capable of causing permanent damage.

Moderate: The effects may cause a deterioration in a patient's clinical status. Additional treatment, hospitalization or extension of hospital stay may be necessary. (Note: an unintended pregnancy resulting from a drug interaction with oral contraceptives is regarded as an interaction of moderate severity.)

Minor: The effects are usually mild; consequences may be bothersome or unnoticeable, but should not significantly affect the therapeutic outcome. Additional treatment is usually not required.

2.2.2 DOCUMENTATION

Documentation is the degree of confidence that an interaction *can* cause an altered clinical response. This scale represents the Editorial Group's evaluation of the quality and clinical relevance of the primary literature supporting the occurrence of an interaction. However, multiple factors can influence whether even a well-documented drug–drug or drug–food interaction occurs in a particular patient. The documentation does not address the incidence or frequency of the interaction; it is also independent of the potential severity of the effect of the interaction.

The following guidelines are used to establish the five Documentation levels:

Established: Proven to occur in well-controlled studies.
- An altered pharmacological effect has been demonstrated in well-controlled human studies ... or ...
- A pharmacokinetic interaction has been demonstrated in well-controlled human studies. An altered pharmacological response is expected based on the magnitude of the kinetic effect; clinical observations also support the occurrence of the interaction.

Probable: Very likely, but not proven clinically.
- A pharmacokinetic interaction has been demonstrated in well-controlled studies. Based on the magnitude of the kinetic changes and the known plasma level–response relationship of the affected drug, an altered pharmacological response will probably occur ... or ...
- When controlled human experimentation is impractical, well-designed animal experiments confirm an interaction which is suggested by multiple case reports or uncontrolled studies.

Suspected: May occur; some good data, but needs more study.
- A pharmacokinetic interaction has been demonstrated in well-controlled studies. Although an altered pharmacological response might be expected to occur based on the magnitude of the kinetic changes, no firm conclusion can be drawn since a plasma level–response relationship has not been established for the affected drug ... or ...
- An altered pharmacologic response has been reported in multiple case reports or repeated uncontrolled clinical studies.

Possible: Could occur, but data are very limited.
- Although a pharmacokinetic interaction has been demonstrated, the kinetic changes are of such magnitude that it is not possible to predict if an altered response will occur ... or ...
- The evidence is divided as to whether an interaction exists ... or ...
- An altered pharmacologic response is suggested by limited data.

Unlikely: Doubtful; no good evidence of an altered clinical effect.
- A pharmacokinetic interaction has been demonstrated; however, based on the magnitude of kinetic change, a pharmacologic alteration is unlikely ... or ...

- The bulk of documentation is of poor quality or does not favor the existence of an interaction ... or ...
- In spite of reports of an interaction, well-controlled studies refute the existence of a clinically relevant interaction.

With regard to the latter documentation level, for the purpose of this review, the authors have chosen to use the qualification 'doubtful documentation level'.

In view of the specific characteristics of the available data on the two types of interactions which may involve oral contraceptives, it is the opinion of the authors that in the product information on oral contraceptives only those interactions are to be included which reach at least both the qualifications 'moderate severity' and 'suspected documentation level'.

Note: Sections 2.2, 2.2.1 and 2.2.2 of this chapter have been reproduced from *Drug Interaction Facts*: © 1993 by Facts and Comparisons. Used with permission from *Drug Interaction Facts. 1993 ed*. St. Louis: Facts and Comparisons, a Division of the J.B. Lippincott Company.

Chapter 3:
Individual Drugs by Pharmacotherapeutic Classification

3.1 β-ADRENERGIC BLOCKERS

Documentation level	*Possible:* No clinical signs of increased β-adrenergic blocker (β-blocker) efficacy or increased incidence of β-blocker-related adverse reactions have been reported. One pharmaco-kinetic interaction study has shown that the area under curve for metoprolol was higher to a statistically significant degree in oral contraceptive users as compared to controls, whereas there were no significant differences in peak plasma concentrations, peak plasma time or elimination half-life between the two groups. The same trend without reaching statistical significance was observed with other oxidatively metabolized β-blockers such as propranolol and oxprenolol, whereas acebutolol (which is metabolized only partly by the liver) showed an opposite trend (Kendall *et al.*, 1982;1984).
Severity	*Minor:* Taking into account the reported magnitude of the above-mentioned changes in the metabolism of β-blockers and the large 'therapeutic window' of this class of drugs, the severity of this drug interaction is probably minor.
Mechanism of action	*Enzyme inhibition:* Both estrogens and progestagens are capable of inhibiting cytochrome P_{450} activity in man (Chambers *et al.*, 1982; Back *et al.*, 1990; Guengerich,1990). Since the β-blockers follow different metabolic pathways, a different effect of oral contraceptive use on β-blocker metabolism can be expected: β-blockers which are oxidized by cytochrome P_{450}-dependent liver enzymes (Guengerich, 1989) may be involved in metabolic drug interactions with oral contraceptives, whereas β-blockers which are excreted unchanged via the kidneys are not. Thus, there are indirect indications for impaired metabolism of oxidatively metabolized β-blockers in oral contraceptive users.
Management	No evidence has been obtained indicating that clinically significant effects occur that would require adjustment of the dose or prescription of an alternative medication.
Clinically significant	No.

References

Back DJ, Houlgrave R, Tjia JF, Ward S, Orme ML'E. Effect of the progestogens, gestodene, 3-ketodesogestrel, levonorgestrel, norethisterone and norgestimate on the oxidation of ethinylestradiol and other substrates by human liver microsome. *J Steroid Biochem Mol Biol* 1991; 38:219–25

Chambers DM, Jefferson GC, Chambers M, Loudon NB. Antipyrine elimination in saliva after low-dose combined or progestogen-only contraceptive steroids. *Br J Clin Pharmacol* 1982;13:229–32

Guengerich FP. Characterization of human microsomal cytochrome P_{450} enzymes. *Ann Rev Pharmacol Toxicol* 1989;29:241–64

Guengerich FP. Mechanism-based inactivation of human liver microsomal cytochrome P_{450}IIIA4 by gestodene. *Chem Res Toxicol* 1990;3:363–71

Kendall MJ, Quarterman CP, Jack DB, Beeley L. Metoprolol pharmacokinetics and the oral contraceptive pill. *Br J Clin Pharmacol* 1982;14:120–2

Kendall MJ, Jack DB, Quarterman CP, *et al*. β-Adrenoceptor blocker pharmacokinetics and the oral contraceptive pill. *Br J Clin Pharmacol* 1984;17:87S–89S

3.2 ADSORBENTS

Documentation level	*Doubtful: In vitro* data indicate that there may be an interaction between adsorbent drugs (antacids, activated charcoal) and oral contraceptives (Khalil and Iwuagdu, 1978; Fadel *et al.*, 1979). However, the only clinical study performed to date has shown that the bioavailability of contraceptive steroids was not impaired in women using antacids concurrently (Joshi *et al.*, 1986). In addition, no cases of contraceptive failure have been attributed to an interaction between oral contraceptives and adsorbents. With regard to activated charcoal and cholestyramine, no reliable human data are available.
Severity	*Moderate:* This interaction is of moderate severity since decreased absorption of contraceptive steroids may result in oral contraceptive failure.
Mechanism of action	*Decreased absorption:* The suggested mechanism of action is that contraceptive efficacy could be impaired when absorption or reabsorption of steroids from the small intestine is inhibited as a result of either impaired direct absorption or impairment of the enterohepatic circulation. This mechanism has been suggested when adsorbents are used concomitantly with oral contraceptives (Ariëns, 1983a,b; Back and Breckenridge, 1978). In this case, contraceptive steroids would attach to the adsorbent agent without dissolving and consequently the steroid would be unable to pass through the gut wall (Ariëns, 1983a,b).
Management	No evidence has been obtained indicating that clinically significant effects occur that would require adjustment of the dose or prescription of an alternative medication.
Clinically significant	No.

References	Ariëns EJ. Actieve kool – "zwarte kunst". *Ned Tijdschr Geneeskd* 1983a;127:592–7
	Ariëns EJ. Actieve Kool Herontdekt. Medische en Farmaceutische Aspecten. *Pharm Weekbl* 1983b; 118:519–33

References

Back DJ, Breckenridge AM. Drug interactions with oral contraceptives. *IPPF Med Bull* 1978;12:1–2

Fadel H, Abd Elbary A, Nour El-Din E, Kassem AA. Availability of norethisterone acetate from combined oral contraceptive tablets. *Pharmazie* 1979;34:49–50

Joshi JV, Sankolli GM, Shah RS, Joshi UM. Antacid does not reduce the bioavailability of oral contraceptive steroids in women. *Int J Clin Pharmacol Ther Toxicol* 1986;24:192–5

Khalil SAH, Iwuagdu M. *In vitro* uptake of oral contraceptive steroids by magnesium trisilicate. *J Pharm Sci* 1978;67:287–9

3.3 ALCOHOL

Documentation level

Doubtful: Some studies indicate that oral contraceptive users experience significantly less impairment of motor test performance during concurrent alcohol use, and also a reduced voluntary alcohol intake as compared to controls (Jones and Jones, 1978; Hobbes *et al.*, 1985). However, these clinical findings are not supported by pharmacokinetic evidence: some studies even showed an impairment of alcohol metabolism (Jones and Jones, 1978; Kegg and Zeiner, 1980; Zeiner and Kegg, 1981; Jones and Jones, 1984), whereas recent studies (with in general a better design) showed no effect of oral contraceptive use on alcohol disposition (Zeiner and Farris, 1979; Hay *et al.*, 1984; Jeavons and Zeiner, 1984; Hobbes *et al.*, 1985; Cole-Harding and Wilson, 1987).

Severity

Minor: Taking into account the reported magnitude of the changes in the metabolism of alcohol as documented in some of the above-mentioned studies, the normal tolerance to alcohol and the severity of this drug interaction (if any) is probably minor.

Mechanism of action

Enzyme inhibition: With regard to the inhibition of alcohol metabolism in connection with oral contraceptive use, two possible mechanisms have been suggested. First, in general, contraceptive steroids have an inhibitory effect on hepatic oxidative metabolism (Chambers *et al.*, 1982; Back *et al.*, 1990; Guengerich, 1990). The isoenzyme responsible for microsomal oxidative alcohol metabolism is cytochrome $P_{450}IIE1$ (Wrighton *et al.*, 1986; Nebert *et al.*, 1989) and this pathway accounts for 10–25% of total alcohol metabolism after single doses (Wrighton *et al.*, 1986). However, the results of the study by Hobbes *et al.* (1985) refute this theory. Second, involvement of the alcohol dehydrogenase pathway (which accounts for 75–90% of total alcohol metabolism after single doses) has been proposed. In agreement with the theory that inhibition of acetaldehyde dehydrogenase may be involved is that in oral contraceptive users, increased acetaldehyde plasma concentration accompanying dysphoric symptoms and decreased voluntary alcohol intake were observed as compared to controls (Jeavons and Zeiner, 1984). However, these findings need to be substantiated further.

Management

No evidence has been obtained indicating that clinically significant effects occur that would require adjustment of the dose or prescription of an alternative medication.

Clinically significant

No.

References

Back DJ, Houlgrave R, Tjia JF, Ward S, Orme ML'E. Effect of the progestogens, gestodene, 3-ketodesogestrel, levonorgestrel, norethisterone and norgestimate on the oxidation of ethinylestradiol and other substrates by human liver microsomes. *J Steroid Biochem Mol Biol 1991; 38:219–25*

Chambers DM, Jefferson GC, Chambers M, Loudon NB. Antipyrine elimination in saliva after low-dose combined or progestogen-only contraceptive steroids. *Br J Clin Pharmacol* 1982;13:229–32

Cole-Harding S, Wilson JR. Ethanol metabolism in men and women. *J Stud Alcohol* 1987;48:380–7

Guengerich FP. Mechanism-based inactivation of human liver microsomal cytochrome $P_{450}IIIA4$ by gestodene. *Chem Res Toxicol* 1990;3:363–71

Hay WM, Nathan PE, Heermans HW, Frankenstein W. Menstrual cycle, tolerance and blood alcohol level discrimination ability. *Addict Behav* 1984;9:67–77

Hobbes J, Boutagy J, Shenfield GM. Interactions between ethanol and oral contraceptive steroids. *Clin Pharmacol Ther* 1985;38:371–80

Jeavons CM, Zeiner AR. Effects of elevated female sex steroids on ethanol and acetaldehyde metabolism in humans. *Alcohol Clin Exp Res* 1984;8:352–8

Jones BM, Jones MK. Interaction of alcohol, oral contraceptives and the menstrual cycle with stimulus–response compatibility. In: Seixas FA, ed. *Currents in Alcoholism*, vol 2. New York: Grune and Stratton, 1978:457–77

Jones MK, Jones BM. Ethanol metabolism in women taking oral contraceptives. *Alcohol Clin Exp Res* 1984;8:24–8

Kegg PS, Zeiner AR. Birth control pill effects on ethanol pharmacokinetics, acetaldehyde and cardiovascular measures in Caucasian females. *Psychophysiology* 1980;17:294

Nebert DW, Nelson DR, Adesnik M, Coon MJ, Estabrook RW, Gonzalez FJ, *et al*. The P_{450} superfamily: updated listing of all genes and recommended nomenclature for the chromosomal loci. *DNA* 1989;8:1–13

References

Wrighton SA, Thomas PE, Molowa DT, Haniu M, Shively JE, Maines SL, *et al.* Characterization of ethanol-inducible human liver *N*-nitrosodimethylamine demethylase. *Biochemistry* 1986;25:6731–5

Zeiner AR, Farris JJ. Male–female and birth control pill effects on ethanol pharmacokinetics in American Indians. *Alcohol Clin Exp Res* 1979;3:202

Zeiner AR, Kegg PS. Menstrual cycle and oral contraceptive effects on alcohol pharmacokinetics in Caucasian females. *Curr Alcohol* 1981;8:47–56

3.4 ANALGESICS

3.4.1 SALICYLATES

Documentation level	*Possible:* There are no reports of clinically significant drug interactions between oral contraceptives and salicylates. Pharmacokinetic drug interaction studies have shown that there may be statistically significant changes in the metabolism of salicylates. In a number of studies, the metabolism of salicylates appeared to be increased in oral contraceptive users as measured by plasma clearance and elimination half-life (Gupta *et al.*, 1982; Miners *et al.*, 1986; 1987; MacDonald *et al.*, 1990).
Severity	*Minor:* Taking into account the reported magnitude of the above-mentioned changes in the metabolism of salicylates and the large 'therapeutic window' of this class of drugs, the severity of this drug interaction is probably minor.
Mechanism of action	*Enzyme induction:* It has been demonstrated that contraceptive steroids are moderate inducers of the uridine diphospho-glucuronosyltransferase enzyme system, whereas other conjugative pathways such as sulfate conjugation are not induced (Miners *et al.*, 1984). Since salicylates are metabolized for the major part via glycine and glucuronide conjugation, it is possible that metabolism of salicylates via this pathway is induced in oral contraceptive users (Hutt *et al.*, 1986; Miners *et al.*, 1986; MacDonald *et al.*, 1990).
Management	No evidence has been obtained indicating that clinically significant effects occur that would require adjustment of the dose or prescription of an alternative medication.
Clinically significant	No.

References	Gupta KC, Joshi JV, Hazari K, *et al.* Effect of low estrogen combination oral contraceptives on metabolism of aspirin and phenylbutazone. *Int J Clin Pharmacol Ther Toxicol* 1982;20: 511–13
	Hutt AJ, Caldwell J, Smith RL. The metabolism of aspirin in man: a population study. *Xenobiotica* 1986;16:239–49
	MacDonald JI, Herman RJ, Verbeeck RK. Sex difference and the effects of smoking and oral contraceptive steroids on the kinetics of diflunisal. *Eur J Clin Pharmacol* 1990;38:175–9

References

Miners JO, Deiner R, Attwood J, Robson R, Birkett DJ. Influence of sex and oral contraceptive steroids on drug glucuronidation. *Clin Exp Pharmacol Physiol* 1984;(Suppl 8):63

Miners JO, Grgurinovich N, Whitehead AG, Robson RA, Birkett DJ. Influence of gender and oral contraceptive steroids on the metabolism of salicylic acid and acetylsalicylic acid. *Br J Clin Pharmacol* 1986;22:135–42

Miners JO, Grgurinovich N, Whitehead AG, Robson RA, Birkett DJ. Influence of gender and oral contraceptive steroids on salicylic acid and acetylsalicylic acid disposition. *Clin Exp Pharmacol Physiol* 1987;(Suppl 10): 22–3

3.4.2 PARACETAMOL
3.4.2a Effect of oral contraceptives on paracetamol pharmacokinetics

Documentation level	*Possible:* There are no reports of a diminished paracetamol efficacy in oral contraceptive users. A number of studies have shown that the metabolism of paracetamol is increased in oral contraceptive users as measured by plasma clearance and elimination half-life (Mucklow *et al.*, 1980; Abernethy *et al.*, 1982; Miners *et al.*, 1983; Mitchell *et al.*, 1983; Ochs *et al.*, 1984; Okonek *et al.*, 1987).
Severity	*Minor:* Taking into account the reported magnitude of the above-mentioned changes in the metabolism of paracetamol and the large 'therapeutic window' of this drug, the severity of this drug interaction is probably minor.
Mechanism of action	*Enzyme induction:* It has been demonstrated that oral contraceptives are moderate inducers of the uridine diphospho-glucuronosyltransferase enzyme system, whereas other conjugative pathways such as sulfate conjugation are not induced (Miners *et al.*, 1984). The induction of the former conjugative pathway was found to be responsible for the increased conjugation of paracetamol in oral contraceptive users (Miners *et al.*, 1983;1990).
Management	No evidence has been obtained indicating that clinically significant effects occur that would require adjustment of the dose or prescription of an alternative medication.
Clinically significant	No.

3.4.2b Effect of paracetamol on oral contraceptive pharmacokinetics

Documentation level	*Possible:* From an *in vitro* study, it appeared that sulfate conjugation of ethinylestradiol in the gastrointestinal mucosa was reduced in the presence of paracetamol (Rogers *et al.*, 1987a). This finding, resulting in enhanced absorption of ethinylestradiol, was supported by an *in vivo* study, showing that the bioavailability of total ethinylestradiol was increased to a statistically significant degree in oral contraceptive users who took paracetamol concurrently as compared to controls. However, the decrease in ethinylestradiol sulfation was compensated for partly by an increase in ethinylestradiol glucuronide conjugation (and thereby leaving free ethinylestradiol plasma concentrations unchanged). The pharmacokinetics of levonorgestrel remained unaffected (Rogers *et al.*, 1987b).

Severity	*Minor:* Taking into account the absence of reports on ethinylestradiol-related side-effects in women using oral contraceptives and paracetamol concurrently, and the large inter- and intraindividual variations in ethinylestradiol plasma levels, the severity of this interaction is probably minor.
Mechanism of action	*Increased absorption:* It was first suggested that this interaction results from competitive enzyme inhibition. However, there is substantial evidence that ethinylestradiol and paracetamol are not substrates for the same sulfotransferase enzyme. Therefore, it is now thought that depletion of the 3'-phosphoadenosine-5'-phosphosulfate pool in the gut wall (the sulfate source in enzymatic sulfation reactions), as a result of consumption by paracetamol conjugation, is responsible for the decreased presystemic ethinylestradiol sulfation and thus increased absorption of ethinylestradiol (Rogers *et al.,* 1987a).
Management	No evidence has been obtained indicating that clinically significant effects occur that would require adjustment of the dose or prescription of an alternative medication.
Clinically significant	No.

References

Abernethy DR, Divoll M, Ochs HR, Ameer B, Greenblatt DJ. Increased metabolic clearance of acetaminophen with oral contraceptive use. *Obstet Gynecol* 1982;60:338–41

Miners JO, Attwood J, Birkett DJ. Influence of sex and oral contraceptive steroids on paracetamol metabolism. *Br J Clin Pharmacol* 1983;16:503–9

Miners JO, Deiner R, Attwood J, Robson R, Birkett DJ. Influence of sex and oral contraceptive steroids on drug glucuronidation. *Clin Exp Pharmacol Physiol* 1984; (Suppl 8): 63

Miners JO, Lillywhite KJ, Yoovathaworn K, Pongmarutai M, Birkett DJ. Characterization of paracetamol UDP-glucuronosyltransferase activity in human liver microsomes. *Biochem Pharmacol* 1990;40:595–600

Mitchell MC, Hanew T, Meredith CG, Schenker S. Effects of oral contraceptive steroids on acetaminophen metabolism and elimination. *Clin Pharmacol Ther* 1983;34:48–53

References

Mucklow JC, Fraser HS, Bulpitt CH, Kahn C, Mould G, Dollery CT. Environmental factors affecting paracetamol metabolism in London factory and office workers. *Br J Clin Pharmacol* 1980;10:67–74

Ochs HR, Greenblatt DJ, Verburg-Ochs B, Abernethy DR, Knüchel M. Differential effects of isoniazid and oral contraceptive steroids on antipyrine oxidation and acetaminophen conjugation. *Pharmacology* 1984;28:188–95

Okonek M, Dittmann M, Bock KW. Paracetamol conjugation: influence of oral contraceptives, old age and liver disease. *Naunyn Schmiedebergs Arch Pharmacol* 1987;335:R104

Rogers SM, Back DJ, Orme ML'E. Intestinal metabolism of ethinylestradiol and paracetamol *in vitro*: studies using Ussing chambers. *Br J Clin Pharmacol* 1987a;23:727–34

Rogers SM, Back DJ, Stevenson PJ, Grimmer SFM, Orme ML'E. Paracetamol interaction with oral contraceptive steroids: increased plasma concentrations of ethinylestradiol. *Br J Clin Pharmacol* 1987b;23:721–5

3.4.3 MORPHINE AND ANALOGS

Documentation level	*Possible:* Although no reports have appeared showing a higher morphine need in oral contraceptive users, it has been shown in a pharmacokinetic drug interaction study that the metabolism of morphine is increased in oral contraceptive users as compared to controls, as measured by increased plasma clearance (Harman *et al.*, 1986; Watson *et al.*, 1986). In another study, oral contraceptive use had no influence on the pharmacokinetics of codeine, a morphine analog (Yue *et al.*, 1989).
Severity	*Minor:* Taking into account the reported magnitude of the above-mentioned changes in the metabolism of morphine and the large 'therapeutic window' of this drug, the severity of this drug interaction is probably minor.
Mechanism of action	*Enzyme induction:* It has been demonstrated that oral contraceptives are moderate inducers of the uridine diphosphoglucuronosyltransferase enzyme system, whereas other conjugative pathways such as sulfate conjugation are not induced (Miners *et al.*, 1984). Since morphine is predominantly metabolized via conjugation into morphine-3-glucuronide and morphine-6-glucuronide (Miners *et al.*, 1988; Hoskin and Hanks, 1990), it is postulated that induction of the uridine diphosphoglucuronosyltransferase conjugative pathway may be responsible for the increased conjugation of morphine in oral contraceptive users (Harman *et al.*, 1986; Watson *et al.*, 1986).
Management	No evidence has been obtained indicating that clinically significant effects occur that would require adjustment of the dose or prescription of an alternative medication.
Clinically significant	No.
References	Harman PJ, Watson KJR, Ghabrial H, Mashford ML, Breen KJ, Desmon PV. Effects of sex and the oral contraceptive pill on morphine disposition. *Acta Pharmacol Toxicol* 1986;59 (Suppl V): 95
	Hoskins PJ, Hanks GW. Morphine: pharmacokinetics and clinical practice. *Br J Cancer* 1990;62:705–7

References

Miners JO, Deiner R, Attwood J, Robson R, Birkett DJ. Influence of sex and oral contraceptive steroids on drug glucuronidation. *Clin Exp Pharmacol Physiol* 1984; (Suppl 8): 63

Miners JO, Lillywhite KJ, Birkett DJ. *In vitro* evidence for the involvement of at least two forms of human liver UDP-glucuronosyltransferase in morphine-3-glucuronidation. *Biochem Pharmacol* 1988;37:2839–45

Watson KJR, Ghabrial H, Mashford ML, Harman PJ, Breen KJ, Desmon PV. The oral contraceptive pill increases morphine clearance but does not increase hepatic blood flow. *Gastroenterology* 1986;90:1779

Yue QY, Svensson JO, Alm C, Sjöquist F, Säwe J. Interindividual and interethnic differences in the demethylation and glucuronidation of codeine. *Br J Clin Pharmacol* 1989;28:629–37

3.4.4 PYRAZOLONE DERIVATIVES

Documentation level

Possible: There are no clinical reports showing an increased efficacy or toxicity of pyrazolone derivatives in oral contraceptive users. Antipyrine (nowadays seldom used because of its severe adverse effects) is almost completely metabolized via cytochrome P_{450}-dependent oxidative metabolism and is used extensively as a model to investigate hepatic metabolizing capacity in man (Abernethy and Greenblatt, 1981). Therefore, many pharmacokinetic drug interaction studies with oral contraceptives have been performed and these studies show unanimously a decrease in plasma clearance and an increase in elimination half-life of antipyrine (O'Malley *et al.*, 1970; Chambers *et al.*, 1982; Teunissen *et al.*, 1982; Scavone *et al.*, 1989; Pazzucconi *et al.*, 1991). Several studies with progestagen-only preparations showed no significant effect on antipyrine metabolism (Chambers *et al.*, 1982; Lundgren *et al.*, 1986). The metabolism of aminopyrine, an antipyrine analog, is also catalyzed by cytochrome P_{450} and its metabolism has also been reported to be inhibited by combined oral contraceptives (Herz *et al.*, 1978; Sonnenberg *et al.*, 1980). However, studies with progestagen-only preparations revealed contradictory results (Herz *et al.*, 1978; Field *et al.*, 1979).

The metabolism of phenylbutazone (O'Malley *et al.*, 1972; Carter *et al.*, 1975; Gupta *et al.*, 1982) does not appear to be inhibited in oral contraceptive users.

With regard to dipyrone (metamizol), findings are contradictory: whereas Bergmann *et al.* (1988) found no interaction, recent data show that, after short-term concurrent use, ethinylestradiol-containing preparations significantly inhibit dipyrone metabolism, but all values return to baseline after prolonged concurrent use (Balogh *et al.*, 1991).

Severity

Minor: Taking into account the reported magnitude of the above-mentioned changes in the metabolism of pyrazolone derivatives, the 'therapeutic window' of this class of drugs and the allergic rather than dose-related origin of severe adverse drug reactions with pyrazolone derivatives (Parker, 1975), the severity of this drug interaction is probably minor.

Mechanism of action

Enzyme inhibition: Both estrogens and progestagens are capable of inhibiting cytochrome P_{450} activity in man (Guengerich, 1990; Back *et al.*, 1991). It appeared that antipyrine metabolism was decreased indicating inhibition of multiple cytochrome P_{450} isoenzymes (Teunissen *et al.*, 1982). The same applies to aminopyrine (Herz *et al.*, 1978) and it is further suggested that specific cytochrome P_{450} isoenzymes that are responsible for biotransformation of phenylbutazone are not induced by oral contraceptive use (Carter *et al.*, 1974;1975). The metabolism of dipyrone probably is inhibited after short-term concurrent oral contraceptive use, the effect disappearing after prolonged concurrent use.

Management	No evidence has been obtained indicating that clinically significant effects occur that would require adjustment of the dose or prescription of an alternative medication.
Clinically significant	No.

References

Abernethy DR, Greenblatt DJ. Impairment of antipyrine metabolism by low-dose oral contraceptive steroids. *Clin Pharmacol Ther* 1981;29:106–10

Back DJ, Houlgrave R, Tjia JF, Ward S, Orme ML'E. Effect of the progestogens, gestodene, 3-ketodesogestrel, levonorgestrel, norethisterone and norgestimate on the oxidation of ethinylestradiol and other substrates by human liver microsomes. *J Steroid Biochem Mol Biol* 1991;38:219–25

Balogh A, Irmisch E, Wolf P, Letrari S, Splinter FK, Hempel E, *et al.* Zum Einfluß von Levonorgestrel und Ethinylestradiol sowie deren Kombination auf die Aktivität von Biotransformationsreaktionen. *Zentralbl Gynaekol* 1991;113:1388–96

Bergmann M, Splinter FC, Henschel L, Balogh A, Hoffmann A, Klinger G. Die Metamizol-Coffein-Elimination bei Frauen mit erhöhten Aminotransferaseaktivitäten im Serum unter steroidalen oralen Kontrazeptiva. *Dtsch Z Verdau Stoffwechselkrankh* 1988;48:261–7

Carter DE, Goldman JM, Bressler R, *et al.* Effect of oral contraceptives on drug metabolism. *Clin Pharmacol Ther* 1974;15:22–31

Carter DE, Bressler R, Hughes MR, *et al.* Effect of oral contraceptives on plasma clearance. *Clin Pharmacol Ther* 1975;18:700–7

Field B, Lu C, Hepner GW. Inhibition of hepatic drug metabolism by norethindrone. *Clin Pharmacol Ther* 1979;25:196–8

References

Guengerich FP. Mechanism-based inactivation of human liver microsomal cytochrome $P_{450}IIIA4$ by gestodene. *Chem Res Toxicol* 1990;3:363–71

Gupta KC, Joshi JV, Hazari K, *et al*. Effect of low estrogen combination oral contraceptive on metabolism of aspirin and phenylbutazone. *Int J Clin Pharmacol Ther Toxicol* 1982;20:511–13

Herz G, Koelz HR, Haemmerti UP, *et al*. Inhibition of hepatic demethylation of aminopyrine by oral contraceptives in humans. *Eur J Clin Invest* 1978;8:27–30

Lundgren S, Kvinnsland S, Utaaker E, Bakke O, Ueland PM. Effect of high-dose progestins on the disposition of antipyrine, digitoxin, and warfarin in patients with advanced breast cancer. *Cancer Chemother Pharmacol* 1986;18:270–5

O'Malley K, Stevenson IH, Alexander W. Increased antipyrine half-life in women taking oral contraceptives. *Scot Med J* 1970;15;454–6

O'Malley K, Stevenson IH, Crooks J. Impairment of human drug metabolism by oral contraceptive steroids. *Clin Pharmacol Ther* 1972;13:552–7

Parker CW. Drug Allergy. *N Engl J Med* 1975;292:511, 732,957

Pazzucconi F, Malavasi B, Galli G, Franceschini G, Calabresi L, Sirtori CR. Inhibition of antipyrine metabolism by low-dose contraceptives with gestodene and desogestrel. *Clin Pharmacol Ther* 1991;49:278–84

Scavone JM, Greenblatt DJ, Abernethy DJ, Luna BG, Harmatz JS. Influence of smoking and oral contraceptive use, alone and together, on antipyrine pharmacokinetics. *J Clin Pharmacol* 1989;29:849

Sonnenberg A, Koelz HR, Herz R, *et al*. Limited usefulness of the breath test in evaluation of drug metabolism: a study in human oral contraceptive users treated with dimethyl-aminoantipyrine and diazepam. *Hepatogastroenterology* 1980;27:104–8

Teunissen MWE, Srivastava AK, Breimer DD. Influence of sex and oral contraceptive steroids on antipyrine metabolite formation. *Clin Pharmacol Ther* 1982;32:240–6

3.4.5 MEPERIDINE (PETHIDINE)

Documentation level	*Doubtful:* Although no reports have been published indicating an enhanced analgesic efficacy of meperidine (pethidine), animal data (Knodell *et al.*, 1982) and a pharmacokinetic drug interaction study in man have shown that the metabolism of the drug was inhibited in oral contraceptive users (Crawford and Rudofsky, 1966). However, these findings are not confirmed by the more sophisticated clinical study by Stambaugh and Wainer (1975) who found no statistically significant impairment of meperidine pharmacokinetics in oral contraceptive users.
Severity	*Minor:* Taking into account the reported magnitude of the above-mentioned changes in the metabolism of meperidine and the 'therapeutic window' of this drug, the severity of this drug interaction (if any) is probably minor.
Mechanism of action	*Enzyme inhibition*: Meperidine is metabolized by cytochrome P_{450}-dependent oxidative metabolism (Edwards *et al.*, 1982), and the increase in urinary excretion of unaltered meperidine was attributed to inhibition of meperidine *N*-demethylation in oral contraceptive users (Crawford and Rudofsky, 1966). However, Stambaugh and Wainer (1975) did not find changes in plasma clearance or changes in meperidine metabolite formation. Thus, evidence is conflicting whether there is a pharmacokinetic drug interaction between oral contraceptives and meperidine and whether enzyme inhibition would be the mechanism of action of such a drug interaction.
Management	No evidence has been obtained indicating that clinically significant effects occur that would require adjustment of the dose or prescription of an alternative medication.
Clinically significant	No.
References	Crawford JS, Rudofsky S. Some alterations in the pattern of drug metabolism associated with pregnancy, oral contraceptives and the newly born. *Br J Anaesth* 1966;38:446–54

References

Edwards DJ, Svensson CK, Visco JP, Lalka D. Clinical pharmacokinetics of pethidine. *Clin Pharmacokinet* 1982;7:421–33

Knodell RG, Allen RC, Kyner WT. Effects of ethinylestradiol on pharmacokinetics of meperidine and pentobarbital in the rat. *J Pharmacol Exp Ther* 1982;221:1–6

Stambaugh JE, Wainer IW. Drug interactions 1: Meperidine and combination oral contraceptives. *J Clin Pharmacol* 1975;15:46–51

3.5 ANTICOAGULANTS

Documentation level

Possible: No cases of increased bleeding tendency or occurrence of thromboembolic events in women using oral contraceptives and anticoagulants concurrently have been reported. Clinical studies have shown contradictory results with regard to drug interactions between oral contraceptives and oral anticoagulants: in one study the clinical response to bishydroxycoumarin was decreased in oral contraceptive users without having any influence on its pharmacokinetic parameters (Schrogie *et al.*, 1967), whereas in another study the clinical response to acenocoumarol was increased in oral contraceptive users but no pharmacokinetic parameters had been investigated (De Teresa *et al.*, 1979). Further, in a recent pharmacokinetic study the metabolism of phenprocoumon was increased to a statistically significant degree in oral contraceptive users as compared to controls as measured by total plasma clearance (Mönig *et al.*, 1990).

With regard to a possible drug interaction between oral contraceptives and the parenterally used anticoagulant heparin, one pharmacokinetic study has indicated that there is no drug interaction between heparin and oral contraceptives (Ence *et al.*, 1976).

Severity

Moderate: Taking into account the reported magnitude of the above-mentioned changes in the metabolism of oral anticoagulants and the 'therapeutic window' of this class of drugs, the severity of this drug interaction is moderate since it is possible that procoagulation may be activated.

Mechanism of action

Enzyme induction/inhibition: It has been demonstrated that oral contraceptives are moderate inducers of the uridine diphosphoglucuronosyltransferase enzyme system (Miners *et al.*, 1984) and inhibitors of cytochrome P_{450}-dependent oxidative metabolism (Back *et al.*, 1990; Guengerich, 1990). Phenprocoumon is metabolized via direct conjugation, but also partly via cytochrome P_{450}-dependent oxidative metabolism. It is suggested that induction of phenprocoumon conjugation by oral contraceptive use is greater than inhibition of its cytochrome P_{450}-dependent oxidative metabolism (Mönig *et al.*, 1990). Other oral anticoagulants such as warfarin and acenocoumarol are metabolized exclusively via oxidative mechanisms (Kaminsky *et al.*, 1984; Thijssen *et al.*, 1986) which suggests that their metabolism would be inhibited in oral contraceptive users, but specific human studies have not been published. However, one animal study with warfarin and contraceptive steroids did not indicate any enzyme inhibition (Roncaglioni *et al.*, 1983).

Management	No evidence has been obtained indicating that clinically significant effects occur that would require adjustment of the dose or prescription of an alternative medication.
Clinically significant	No.

References

Back DJ, Houlgrave R, Tjia JF, Ward S, Orme ML'E. Effect of the progestogens, gestodene, 3-ketodesogestrel, levonorgestrel, norethisterone and norgestimate on the oxidation of ethinylestradiol and other substrates by human liver microsomes. *J Steroid Biochem Mol Biol* 1991;38:219–25

De Teresa E, Vera A, Ortigosa J, *et al*. Interaction between anticoagulants and contraceptives: an unsuspected finding. *Br Med J* 1979;2:1260–1

Ence TJ, Wilson DE, Flowers CM, Chen AL, Glad BW, Hershgold EJ. Heparin metabolism and heparin-released lipase activity during long-term estrogen–progestin treatment. *Metabolism* 1976;25:139–45

Guengerich FP. Mechanism-based inactivation of human liver microsomal cytochrome $P_{450}IIIA4$ by gestodene. *Chem Res Toxicol* 1990;3:363–71

Kaminsky LS, Dunbar DA, Wang PP, *et al*. Human hepatic cytochrome P_{450} composition as probed by *in vitro* microsomal metabolism of warfarin. *Drug Metab Disp* 1984;12:470–7

Miners JO, Deiner R, Attwood J, Robson R, Birkett DJ. Influence of sex and oral contraceptive steroids on drug glucuronidation. *Clin Exp Pharmacol Physiol* 1984;(Suppl 8):63

Mönig H, Baese C, Heidemann HT, Ohnhaus EE, Schulte HM. Effect of oral contraceptive steroids on the pharmacokinetics of phenprocoumon. *Br J Clin Pharmacol* 1990;30:115–18

References

Roncaglioni MC, Gerna M, Wiezowska B, Latini R, Donati MB. Interaction between warfarin and a steroidal contraceptive combination: evidence from a rat model. *Thromb Haemost* 1983;50:303

Schrogie JJ, Solomon HM, Zieve PD. Effect of oral contraceptives on vitamin K-dependent clotting activity. *Clin Pharmacol Ther* 1967;8:670–5

Thijssen HHW, Janssen GMJ, Baars LGM. Lack of effect of cimetidine on pharmacodynamics and kinetics of single oral doses of R- and S-acenocoumarol. *Eur J Clin Pharmacol* 1986;30:619–23

3.6 ANTICONVULSANTS

3.6.1 PHENYTOIN

Documentation level	*Established:* At least 50 pregnancies have been reported in the literature (Organon literature search, 1992). In addition, a recent pharmacokinetic interaction study showed that phenytoin decreased the area under curve of both ethinylestradiol and levonorgestrel (Crawford *et al.*, 1989;1990).
Severity	*Moderate:* This interaction is of moderate severity since the increased metabolism of contraceptive steroids may result in oral contraceptive failure.
Mechanism of action	*Enzyme induction*: In the antipyrine clearance test it has been shown that phenytoin is a potent enzyme inducer (Perucca *et al.*, 1984). The major metabolic pathway of ethinylestradiol is 2-hydroxylation by cytochrome P_{450}IIIA4 (Guengerich, 1988) and it has recently been shown that this enzyme subfamily is inducible by phenytoin (Ball *et al.*, 1990).
Management	(1) An alternative drug without enzyme-inducing properties should be used.

Management (continued):

(2) In the case of long-term concurrent enzyme-inducing drug treatment:

- It is recommended to prescribe as a standard starting routine a monophasic 50 µg ethinylestradiol oral contraceptive (do not prescribe an oral contraceptive with placebo tablets, every-day pill).
- For example, the dosage regimen with this oral contraceptive could be four packs in a row followed by a tablet-free interval of 5 or 6 days.
- The contraceptive efficacy of the regimen can be judged on the basis of the occurrence of irregular bleeding (IB). IB is reviewed normally during the first follow-up visit (i.e. after the first four packs have been used). However, the woman should be advised that if IB is heavy and prolonged she should return sooner.
- If IB is too frequent:
  - Increase the ethinylestradiol dose either by using a regimen of two sub-50 µg ethinylestradiol oral contraceptive tablets/day (i.e. 2 tablets with 30–35 µg ethinylestradiol/tablet) or a regimen of one 50 µg ethinylestradiol oral contraceptive tablet + one sub-50 µg ethinylestradiol oral contraceptive tablet/day.
  - If IB still continues, increase the ethinylestradiol dose further to two 50 µg ethinylestradiol oral contraceptive tablets/day.

- If the above options are still not successful in controlling IB, use of an alternative contraceptive method should be advised.

Note that after enzyme-inducing medication has been stopped, liver enzyme induction may be sustained during a period of approximately 4 weeks. Therefore, during this period, it is necessary either to stay on the higher dose oral contraceptive regimen or, when the woman resumes low-dose oral contraceptive use, in addition, to use a barrier method.

Clinically significant	Yes.

References

Ball SE, Forrester LM, Wolf CR, Back DJ. Differences in the cytochrome P_{450} isozymes involved in the 2-hydroxylation of estradiol and 17α-ethinylestradiol: relative activities of rat and human liver enzymes. *Biochem J* 1990;267:221–6

Crawford P, Chadwick D, Cleland P, *et al*. Oral contraceptive steroids and anticonvulsant therapy. *4th International Symposium on Sodium Valproate and Epilepsy*, 27th April 1989, Jersey. Abstracts. 1989:82

Crawford P, Chadwick DJ, Martin C, Tjia J, Back DJ, Orme M. The interaction of phenytoin and carbamazepine with combined oral contraceptive steroids. *Br J Clin Pharmacol* 1990;30:892–6

Guengerich FP. Oxidation of 17α-ethinylestradiol by human liver cytochrome P_{450}. *Mol Pharmacol* 1988;33:500–8

Perucca E, Hedges A, Makki KA, Ruprah M, Wilson JF, Richens A. A comparative study of the relative enzyme inducing properties of anticonvulsant drugs in epileptic patients. *Br J Clin Pharmacol* 1984;18:401–10

3.6.2 BARBITURATES

Documentation level	*Established:* At least 50 pregnancies have been reported in the literature (Organon literature search,1992). Pharmacokinetic data have shown that plasma levels of ethinylestradiol are reduced in women using oral contraceptives and barbiturates concurrently (Back *et al.*, 1980a; Crawford *et al.*, 1989). In one of these studies, total norethisterone levels remained unaffected but there was a significant increase in sex hormone binding globulin which effectively reduces the free norethisterone plasma levels (Back *et al.*, 1980a). However, the clinical relevance of this finding remains to be shown.
Severity	*Moderate:* This interaction is of moderate severity since the increased metabolism of contraceptive steroids may result in oral contraceptive failure.
Mechanism of action	*Enzyme induction:* In the antipyrine clearance test, it was shown that phenobarbital is a potent enzyme inducer (Perucca *et al.*, 1984). The major metabolic pathway of ethinylestradiol is 2-hydroxylation by cytochrome $P_{450}IIIA4$ (Guengerich, 1988) and it has been shown recently that this enzyme subfamily is inducible by phenobarbital (Ball *et al.*, 1990). In addition, enzyme-inducing drugs are known to increase sex hormone binding globulin binding capacity (Victor *et al.*, 1977; Back *et al.*, 1980b).

Management	(1) An alternative drug without enzyme-inducing properties should be used.
	
	(2) In the case of long-term concurrent enzyme-inducing drug treatment:
	– It is recommended to prescribe as a standard starting routine a monophasic 50 µg ethinylestradiol oral contraceptive (do not prescribe an oral contraceptive with placebo tablets, every-day pill).
	– For example, the dosage regimen with this oral contraceptive could be four packs in a row followed by a tablet-free interval of 5 or 6 days.
	– The contraceptive efficacy of the regimen can be judged on the basis of the occurrence of irregular bleeding (IB). IB is reviewed normally during the first follow-up visit (i.e. after the first four packs have been used). However, the woman should be advised that if IB is heavy and prolonged she should return sooner.
	  – If IB is too frequent:
	  • Increase the ethinylestradiol dose either by using a regimen of two sub-50 µg ethinylestradiol oral contra-

ceptive tablets/day (i.e. 2 tablets with 30–35 µg ethinylestradiol/tablet) or a regimen of one 50 µg ethinylestradiol oral contraceptive tablet + one sub-50 µg ethinylestradiol oral contraceptive tablet/day.

- If IB still continues, increase the ethinylestradiol dose further to two 50 µg ethinylestradiol oral contraceptive tablets/day.

- If the above options are still not successful in controlling IB, the use of an alternative contraceptive method should be advised.

Note that after enzyme-inducing medication has been stopped, liver enzyme induction may be sustained during a period of approximately 4 weeks. Therefore, during this period, it is necessary either to stay on the higher dose oral contraceptive regimen or, when the woman resumes low-dose oral contraceptive use, in addition, to use a barrier method.

Clinically significant	Yes.

References	Back DJ, Bates M, Bowden A, *et al*. The interaction of phenobarbital and other anticonvulsants with oral contraceptive steroid therapy. *Contraception* 1980a;22:495–503
	Back DJ, Breckenridge AM, Crawford FE, *et al*. The effect of oral contraceptive steroids and enzyme inducing drugs on sex hormone binding globulin capacity in women. *Br J Clin Pharmacol* 1980b; 9:115
	Ball SE, Forrester LM, Wolf CR, Back DJ, Differences in the cytochrome P_{450} isozymes involved in the 2-hydroxylation of estradiol and 17α-ethinylestradiol: relative activities of rat and human liver enzymes. *Biochem J* 1990;267:221–6
	Crawford P, Chadwick D, Cleland P, *et al*. Oral contraceptive steroids and anticonvulsant therapy. *4th International Symposium on Sodium Valproate and Epilepsy*, 27th April 1989, Jersey. Abstracts. 1989;82
	Guengerich FP. Oxidation of 17α-ethinylestradiol by human liver cytochrome P_{450}. *Mol Pharmacol* 1988;33:500–8
	Perucca E, Hedges A, Makki KA, Ruprah M, Wilson JF, Richens A. A comparative study of the relative enzyme inducing properties of anticonvulsant drugs in epileptic patients. *Br J Clin Pharmacol* 1984;18:401–10
	Victor A, Lundberg PO, Johansson EDB. Induction of sex hormone binding globulin by phenytoin. *Br Med J* 1977;2:934–5

3.6.3 CARBAMAZEPINE

Documentation level

Established: At least 25 pregnancies have been reported in the literature (Organon literature search, 1992). In addition, a recent pharmacokinetic interaction study showed that carbamazepine decreased the area under curve of both ethinylestradiol and levonorgestrel (Crawford *et al.*, 1989;1990).

Severity

Moderate: This interaction is of moderate severity since the increased metabolism of contraceptive steroids may result in oral contraceptive failure.

Mechanism of action

Enzyme induction: In the antipyrine clearance test it has been shown that carbamazepine is a potent enzyme inducer (Perucca *et al.*, 1984). The major metabolic pathway of ethinylestradiol is 2-hydroxylation by cytochrome $P_{450}IIIA4$ (Guengerich, 1988) and it is thought that (similar to pheno-barbital and phenytoin) this enzyme subfamily is inducible by carbamazepine.

Management

(1) An alternative drug without enzyme-inducing properties should be used.

(2) In the case of long-term concurrent enzyme-inducing drug treatment:

– It is recommended to prescribe as a standard starting routine a monophasic 50 µg ethinylestradiol oral contra-ceptive (do not prescribe an oral contraceptive with placebo tablets, every-day pill).

– For example, the dosage regimen with this oral contra-ceptive could be four packs in a row followed by a tablet-free interval of 5 or 6 days.

– The contraceptive efficacy of the regimen can be judged on the basis of the occurrence of irregular bleeding (IB). IB is reviewed normally during the first follow-up visit (i.e. after the first four packs have been used). However, the woman should be advised that if IB is heavy and prolonged she should return sooner.

– If IB is too frequent:

• Increase the ethinylestradiol dose either by using a regimen of two sub-50 µg ethinylestradiol oral contra-ceptive tablets/day (i.e. 2 tablets with 30–35 µg ethinylestradiol/tablet) or a regimen of one 50 µg ethinylestradiol oral contraceptive tablet + one sub-50 µg ethinylestradiol oral contraceptive tablet/day.

- If IB still continues, increase the ethinylestradiol dose further to two 50 µg ethinylestradiol oral contraceptive tablets/day.
- If the above options are still not successful in controlling IB, the use of an alternative contraceptive method should be advised.

Note that after enzyme-inducing medication has been stopped, liver enzyme induction may be sustained during a period of about 4 weeks. Therefore, during this period, it is necessary either to stay on the higher dose oral contraceptive regimen or, when the woman resumes low-dose oral contraceptive use, in addition, to use a barrier method.

Clinically significant	Yes.

References

Crawford P, Chadwick D, Cleland P, *et al*. Oral contraceptive steroids and anticonvulsant therapy. *4th International Symposium on Sodium Valproate and Epilepsy*, 27th April 1989, Jersey. Abstracts. 1989;82

Crawford P, Chadwick DJ, Martin C, Tjia J, Back DJ, Orme M. The interaction of phenytoin and carbamazepine with combined oral contraceptive steroids. *Br J Clin Pharmacol* 1990;30:892–6

Guengerich FP. Oxidation of 17α-ethinylestradiol by human liver cytochrome P_{450}. *Mol Pharmacol* 1988;33:500–8

Perucca E, Hedges A, Makki KA, Ruprah M, Wilson JF, Richens A. A comparative study of the relative enzyme inducing properties of anticonvulsant drugs in epileptic patients. *Br J Clin Pharmacol* 1984;18:401–10

3.6.4 SODIUM VALPROATE

Documentation level	*Doubtful:* Although five pregnancies have been reported in the literature (Organon literature search, 1992), it is assumed that these pregnancies must be attributed to other anticonvulsants which had been used concurrently with sodium valproate in oral contraceptive users. In addition, a recent pharmacokinetic interaction study showed that sodium valproate has no influence on the area under curve of both ethinylestradiol and levonorgestrel (Back and Orme, 1990; Crawford *et al.*, 1989).
Severity	*Not applicable:* There is probably no drug interaction between oral contraceptives and valproic acid.
Mechanism of action	*No mechanism:* In the antipyrine clearance test, it was shown that sodium valproate has no enzyme-inducing properties since the substance did not differ from controls (Perucca *et al.*, 1984). Also in other experiments it appeared that sodium valproate was not an enzyme inducer (Jordan *et al.*, 1976; Oxley *et al.*, 1979).
Management	No evidence has been obtained indicating that clinically significant effects occur which would require adjustment of the dose or prescription of an alternative medication.
Clinically significant	No.

References

Back DJ, Orme ML'E. Pharmacokinetic drug interactions with oral contraceptives. *Clin Pharmacokinet* 1990;18:472–84

Crawford P, Chadwick D, Cleland P, *et al*. Oral contraceptive steroids and anticonvulsant therapy. *4th International Symposium on Sodium Valproate and Epilepsy*, 27th April 1989, Jersey, Abstracts. 1989;82

Jordan BJ, Shillingford JS, Steed KP. Preliminary observations on the protein-binding and enzyme-inducing properties of sodium valproate. In: Legg NJ, ed. *Clinical and Pharmacological Aspects of Sodium Valproate (Epilim) in the Treatment of Epilepsy*. Tunbridge Wells: MCS Consultants,1976:112–16

References   Oxley J, Hedges A, Makki KA, *et al*. A lack of hepatic enzyme inducing effect of sodium valproate. *Br J Clin Pharmacol* 1979;8:189–90

Perucca E, Hedges A, Makki KA, Ruprah M, Wilson JF, Richens A. A comparative study of the relative enzyme inducing properties of anticonvulsant drugs in epileptic patients. *Br J Clin Pharmacol* 1984;18:401–10

3.6.5 ETHOSUXIMIDE

Documentation level	*Doubtful:* Although five pregnancies have been reported in the literature (Organon literature search, 1992), it is assumed that these pregnancies must be attributed to other anticonvulsants which had been used concurrently with ethosuximide in oral contraceptive users.
Severity	*Not applicable:* There is probably no drug interaction between oral contraceptives and ethosuximide.
Mechanism of action	*No mechanism:* There are indications that suximides do not have enzyme-inducing properties which could lead to clinically significant drug interactions (Gilbert *et al.*, 1974; Kutt, 1984).
Management	No evidence has been obtained indicating that clinically significant effects occur that would require adjustment of the dose or prescription of an alternative medication.
Clinically significant	No.

References	Gilbert JC, Scott AK, Galloway DB, Petrie JC. Ethosuximide: liver enzyme induction and D-glucaric acid excretion. *Br J Clin Pharmacol* 1974;1:249–52
	Kutt H. Interactions between anticonvulsants and other commonly prescribed drugs. *Epilepsia* 1984;25:S118–31

3.7 ANTIDEPRESSANTS

Documentation level	*Possible:* In one study, signs of an increased antidepressant efficacy have been observed during the concurrent use of oral contraceptives and imipramine (Prange *et al.*, 1972). In a number of studies in which clomipramine and oral contraceptives have been used concurrently, neither increased clomipramine efficacy nor increased incidence of adverse drug reactions has been observed (Beaumont, 1973; Gringras *et al.*, 1980; John *et al.*, 1980; Luscombe and John, 1980; Seldrup, 1980). Pharmacokinetic drug interaction studies show a similar picture: imipramine bioavailability is increased and plasma clearance is decreased in oral contraceptive users as compared to controls (Abernethy *et al.*, 1984), whereas during the use of clomipramine, there are no pharmacokinetic changes as compared to controls (John *et al.*, 1980; Luscombe and John, 1980; Seldrup, 1980). Similar to imipramine, the metabolism of amitriptyline seems also to be inhibited during the concurrent use of oral contraceptives (Edelbroek *et al.*, 1987).
Severity	*Minor:* Taking into account the reported magnitude of the above-mentioned changes in the metabolism of antidepressants and the large 'therapeutic window' of this class of drugs, the severity of this drug interaction is probably minor.
Mechanism of action	*Enzyme inhibition:* Oral contraceptives are reported to inhibit hepatic microsomal enzymes which metabolize drugs by oxidative processes (Tephly and Mannering, 1968; Mackinnon *et al.*, 1977), which is also the main metabolic pathway for antidepressants (Crome and Dawling, 1989; Sallee and Pollock, 1990). The tricyclic antidepressant drugs amitriptyline, clomipramine, desipramine, imipramine and nortriptyline are oxidized predominantly by cytochrome $P_{450}IID6$ (Guengerich, 1989; Brosen, 1990), an isoenzyme which has been shown to be inhibited by contraceptive steroids (Kallio *et al.*, 1988). Presumably, this enzyme also plays a role in the oxidation of most of the other tricyclic antidepressant drugs. The absence of a drug interaction between oral contraceptives and clomipramine remains to be explained.
Management	No evidence has been obtained indicating that clinically significant effects occur that would require adjustment of the dose or prescription of an alternative medication.
Clinically significant	No.

References

Abernethy DR, Greenblatt DJ, Shader RI. Imipramine disposition in users of oral contraceptive steroids. *Clin Pharmacol Ther* 1984;35:792–7

Beaumont G. Drug interactions with clomipramine (Anafranil). *J Int Med Res* 1973;1:480–4

Brosen K. Recent developments in hepatic drug oxidation – implications for clinical pharmacokinetics. *Clin Pharmacokinet* 1990;18:220–39

Crome P, Dawling S. Pharmacokinetics of tricyclic and related antidepressants. In: Ghose K, ed. *Antidepressants for Elderly People.* London: Chapman and Hall, 1989:117–36

Edelbroek PM, Zitman FG, Knoppert-van der Klein EAM, Putten PM van, Wolff FA de. Therapeutic drug monitoring of amitriptyline: impact of age, smoking and oral contraceptives on drug and metabolic levels in bulimic women. *Clin Chim Acta* 1987;165:177–87

Gringras M, Beaumont G, Grieve A. Clomipramine and oral contraceptives: an interaction study–clinical findings. *J Int Med Res* 1980;8 (Suppl 3):76–80

Guengerich FP. Characterization of human microsomal cytochrome P_{450} enzymes. *Ann Rev Pharmacol Toxicol* 1989;29:241–64

John VA, Luscombe DK, Kemp H. Effects of age, cigarette smoking and the contraceptive pill on the pharmacokinetics of clomipramine and its desmethyl metabolite during chronic dosing. *J Int Med Res* 1980;8 (Suppl 3):88–95

Kallio J, Lindberg R, Huupponen R, IIsalo E. Debrisoquine oxidation in a Finnish population: the effect of oral contraceptives on the metabolic ratio. *Br J Clin Pharmacol* 1988;26:791–5

Luscombe DK, John V. Influence of age, cigarette smoking and the oral contraceptive on plasma concentrations of clomipramine. *Postgrad Med J* 1980;56 (Suppl 1): 99–102

Mackinnon M, Sutherland E, Simon FE. Effects of ethinylestradiol on hepatic microsomal proteins and the turnover of cytochrome P_{450}. *J Lab Clin Med* 1977;90: 1096–106

References

Prange AJ, Wilson IC, Alltop LB. Estrogens may well affect response to antidepressant. *J Am Med Assoc* 1972;219:143–4

Sallee FR, Pollock BG. Clinical pharmacokinetics of imipramine and desipramine. *Clin Pharmacokinet* 1990;18: 346–64

Seldrup J. Relating plasma levels of clomipramine and clinical response. *J Int Med Res* 1980;8 (Suppl 3):96–110

Tephly TR, Mannering GJ. Inhibition of drug metabolism. *Mol Pharmacol* 1968;4:10–14

3.8 ANTIHISTAMINES (H$_1$ AND H$_2$ ANTAGONISTS)

3.8a Effects of oral contraceptives on antihistamine pharmacokinetics

Documentation level	*Doubtful:* There are no clinical reports indicating that oral contraceptive use might interfere with antihistamine efficacy. In addition, from pharmacokinetic studies it appeared that oral contraceptive use did not interfere with the pharmacokinetics of the H$_1$ antagonists doxylamine and diphenhydramine (Luna *et al.*, 1989) and did not also interfere with the drug disposition of the H$_2$ antagonist, cimetidine (Grahnén *et al.*, 1979).
Severity	*Minor:* Taking into account the reported magnitude of the above-mentioned changes in the metabolism of both H$_1$ and H$_2$ antagonists and the large 'therapeutic window' of these classes of drugs, the severity of these drug interactions (if any) is probably minor.
Mechanism of action	*Enzyme inhibition:* Although both estrogens and progestagens are capable of inhibiting cytochrome P$_{450}$ activity in man (Chambers *et al.*, 1982; Back *et al.*, 1990; Guengerich, 1990), the above studies indicate that oral contraceptive use does not inhibit the cytochrome P$_{450}$ families involved in the metabolism of H$_1$ and H$_2$ antagonists.
Management	No evidence has been obtained indicating that clinically significant effects occur that would require adjustment of the dose or prescription of an alternative medication.
Clinically significant	No.

3.8b Effect of antihistamines on oral contraceptive pharmacokinetics

Documentation level	*Doubtful:* Although four pregnancies allegedly due to the concurrent use of oral contraceptives and H$_1$ antagonists have been reported in the literature (DeSano and Hurley, 1982), three of these cases can be probably attributed to concurrently administered antibiotics, whereas the fourth oral contraceptive-associated pregnancy remains unexplained. No reports of impaired contraceptive efficacy during the concurrent use of H$_2$ antagonists and oral contraceptives have been published.

Severity	*Moderate:* This interaction is of moderate severity since the increased metabolism of contraceptive steroids may result in oral contraceptive failure.
Mechanism of action	*Enzyme induction/enzyme inhibition:* Recently, a UK Expert Committee has concluded that phenothiazine-derived H_1 antagonists have no enzyme-inducing properties in man and therefore are probably not capable of impairing oral contraceptive efficacy (CSAC, 1989a,b). Also, with regard to other H_1 antagonists, no evidence is available that they may impair oral contraceptive efficacy. The H_2 antagonist, cimetidine, did not inhibit the cytochrome P_{450}-dependent biotransformation of desogestrel to 3-ketodesogestrel (Madden et al., 1990). In addition, the absence of an effect of H_2 antagonists on oral contraceptive biotransformation was demonstrated further by Meyer *et al.* (1987) who showed that use of roxatidine did not impair oral contraceptive-induced ovulatory suppression.
Management	No evidence has been obtained indicating that clinically significant effects occur that would require adjustment of the dose or prescription of an alternative medication.
Clinically significant	No.

References	Back DJ, Houlgrave R, Tjia JF, Ward S, Orme ML'E. Effect of the progestogens, gestodene, 3-ketodesogestrel, levonorgestrel, norethisterone and norgestimate on the oxidation of ethinylestradiol and other substrates by human liver microsomes. *J Steroid Biochem Mol Biol* 1991;38:219–25
	Chambers DM, Jefferson GC, Chambers M, Loudon NB. Antipyrine elimination in saliva after low-dose combined or progestogen-only contraceptive steroids. *Br J Clin Pharmacol* 1982;13:229–32
	CSAC (Clinical and Scientific Advisory Committee of the National Association of Family Planning Doctors). The COC and phenothiazines. *Br J Fam Plan* 1989a;15:26
	CSAC (Clinical and Scientific Advisory Committee of the National Association of Family Planning Doctors). Drug interaction with enzyme-inducing drugs. *Br J Fam Plan* 1989b;15:65

References

DeSano EA, Hurley SC. Possible interactions of antihist-amines and antibiotics with oral contraceptive effectiveness. *Fertil Steril* 1982;37:853–4

Grahnén A, Bahr C von, Lindström B, Rosén A. Bioavailability and pharmacokinetics of cimetidine. *Eur J Clin Pharmacol* 1979;16:335–40

Guengerich FP. Mechanism-based inactivation of human liver microsomal cytochrome P_{450}IIIA4 by gestodene. *Chem Res Toxicol* 1990;3:363–71

Luna BG, Scavone JM, Greenblatt DJ. Doxylamine and diphenhydramine pharmacokinetics in women on low-dose estrogen oral contraceptives. *J Clin Pharmacol* 1989;29:257–60

Madden S, Back DJ, Orme ML'E. Metabolism of the contra-ceptive steroid desogestrel by human liver *in vitro*. *J Steroid Biochem* 1990;35:281–8

Meyer BH, Müller FO, Luus H, Wessels P, Badian M, Röthig H-J. A model to investigate interactions obtunding oral con-traceptive activity. *Med Sci Res* 1987;15:1497

3.9 ANTIMICROBIALS

3.9.1 PENICILLIN AND DERIVATIVES

Documentation level	*Probable:* Contradictory findings exist. At least 120 pregnancies have been reported in the literature, the number being very small in view of the extensive use of oral contraceptives (Organon literature search, 1992). In controlled clinical studies, penicillins do not interfere with oral contraceptive efficacy as measured by pharmacodynamic and/or pharmacokinetic parameters (Friedman *et al.*, 1980; Joshi *et al.*, 1980; Back *et al.*, 1982). A small retrospective study is suggestive of an increased risk of pill failure in women using certain antibiotics and oral contraceptives concurrently (Hughes and Cunliffe, 1990). However, considering its obvious flaws, it is questionable whether firm conclusions can be drawn from this study (De Groot *et al.*, 1991).
Severity	*Moderate:* This interaction is of moderate severity since the increased metabolism of contraceptive steroids may result in oral contraceptive failure.
Mechanism of action	*Disturbance of the enterohepatic circulation:* It is concluded that oral contraceptive failure associated with concurrent use of certain antibiotics probably results from the coincidence of a number of factors that alter the enterohepatic circulation of ethinylestradiol. These include:

(1) Relatively low ethinylestradiol bioavailability due to extensive gut wall metabolism;

(2) A gut flora which is not capable of adequately hydrolyzing ethinlylestradiol conjugates; and

(3) A gut flora which is susceptible to the activity of the antimicrobial concerned.

It is postulated that the co-occurrence of these phenomena only takes place in certain individuals and that therefore the above-mentioned studies have failed to show any systematic interaction between oral contraceptives and certain antibiotics (including penicillins) (Back and Orme, 1990).

In animals, progestagens undergo enterohepatic circulation only as inactive metabolites, since the unchanged drug cannot be conjugated directly (Back *et al.*, 1978). Therefore, disturbance of the enterohepatic circulation plays no role here. These animal findings are supported by human studies in which no statistically significant effects on pharmacokinetic parameters of levonorgestrel (Back *et al.*, 1982) and norethisterone (Joshi *et al.*, 1980b) were observed in long-term oral contraceptive users during ampicillin treatment.

Management

In the case of short-term concurrent drug treatment, a barrier method should be used both during concurrent drug therapy and for 7 days after discontinuation. If this would continue into the next oral contraceptive tablet-free interval, the woman should skip the tablet-free interval and start the next pack as soon as she has finished the pack in use.

Clinically significant

Yes.

References

Back DJ, Breckenridge AM, Challiner M, *et al*. The effect of antibiotics on the enterohepatic circulation of ethinylestradiol and norethisterone in the rat. *J Steroid Biochem* 1978;9:527–31

Back DJ, Breckenridge AM, MacIver M, *et al*. The effects of ampicillin on oral contraceptive steroids in women. *Br J Clin Pharmacol* 1982; 14:43–8

Back DJ, Orme ML'E Pharmacokinetic drug interactions with oral contraceptives. *Clin Pharmacokinet* 1990;18:472–84

Friedman CI, Huneke AL, Kim MH, Powell J. The effect of ampicillin on oral contraceptive effectiveness. *Obstet Gynecol* 1980;55:33–7

Groot AC De, Eshuis H, Stricker BHC. Oral contraceptives and antibiotics in acne. *Br J Dermatol* 1991; 124:212

Hughes BR, Cunliffe WJ. Interactions between the oral contraceptive pill and antibiotics. *Br J Dermatol* 1990;122:717–18

Joshi JV, Joshi VM, Sankholi GM, *et al*. A study of inter-action of low-dose combination oral contraceptive with ampicillin and metronidazole. *Contraception* 1980b;22:643–52

3.9.2 TETRACYCLINES

Documentation level

Probable: Contradictory findings exist. At least 40 pregnancies have been reported in the literature, the number being very small in view of the extensive use of oral contraceptives (Organon literature search, 1992). In a small study it was indicated that there was a shift from urinary to fecal excretion of tetracycline in oral contraceptive users which points to a disturbed enterohepatic circulation (Swenson et al., 1980; Hudson and Callen, 1982). In contrast, the concurrent use of oral contraceptives and tetracycline in acne patients did not result in a statistically significant decrease of ethinylestradiol or levonorgestrel plasma levels during antibiotic treatment (Orme and Back, 1986). In other drug interaction studies with tetracycline (Murphy et al., 1991) and its derivative doxycycline (Neely et al., 1991), the concurrent use of a combined low-dose oral contraceptive did not result in altered plasma concentrations of norethisterone, ethinylestradiol or endogenous progesterone as compared to control subjects.

A small retrospective study is suggestive of an increased risk of pill failure in women using certain antibiotics and oral contraceptives concurrently (Hughes and Cunliffe, 1990). However, considering its obvious flaws, it is questionable whether firm conclusions can be drawn from this study (De Groot et al., 1991).

Severity

Moderate: This interaction is of moderate severity since the increased metabolism of contraceptive steroids may result in oral contraceptive failure.

Mechanism of action

Disturbance of the enterohepatic circulation: It is concluded that oral contraceptive failure associated with concurrent use of certain antibiotics probably results from the coincidence of a number of factors that alter the enterohepatic circulation of ethinylestradiol. These include:

(1) Relatively low ethinylestradiol absorption capacity due to extensive gut wall metabolism;

(2) A gut flora which is not capable of adequately hydrolyzing ethinlylestradiol conjugates; and

(3) A gut flora which is susceptible to the activity of the antimicrobial concerned.

It is postulated that the co-occurrence of these phenomena only takes place in certain individuals and that, therefore, the above-mentioned studies have failed to show any systematic interaction between oral contraceptives and certain antibiotics (including tetracyclines) (Back and Orme, 1990).

In animals, progestagens undergo enterohepatic circulation only as inactive metabolites, since the unchanged drug cannot be conjugated directly (Back *et al.*, 1978). Therefore, disturbance of the enterohepatic circulation plays no role here. These animal findings are supported by human studies in which no statistically significant effects on pharmacokinetic parameters of norethisterone (Murphy *et al.*, 1991; Neely *et al.*, 1991) were observed in long-term oral contraceptive users during treatment with tetracycline or doxycycline.

Management	In the case of short-term concurrent drug treatment, a barrier method should be used both during concurrent drug treatment and for 7 days after discontinuation. If this would continue into the next oral contraceptive tablet-free interval, the woman should skip the tablet-free interval and start the next pack as soon as she has finished the pack in use.
Clinically significant	Yes.

References

Back DJ, Breckenridge AM, Challiner M, *et al*. The effect of antibiotics on the enterohepatic circulation of ethinylestradiol and norethisterone in the rat. *J Steroid Biochem* 1978;9:527–31

Back DJ, Orme ML'E. Pharmacokinetic drug interactions with oral contraceptives. *Clin Pharmacokinet* 1990;18:472–84

Groot AC De, Eshuis H, Stricker BHC. Oral contraceptives and antibiotics in acne. *Br J Dermatol* 1991; 124:212

Hudson CP, Callen JP. The tetracycline–oral contraceptive controversy. *J Am Acad Dermatol* 1982;7:269–70

Hughes BR, Cunliffe WJ. Interactions between the oral contraceptive pill and antibiotics. *Br J Dermatol* 1990;122:717–18

Murphy AA, Zacur HA, Charache P, Burkman RT. The effect of tetracycline on levels of oral contraceptives. *Am J Obstet Gynecol* 1991;164:28–33

Neely JL, Abate M, Swinker M, D'Angio R. The effect of doxycycline on serum levels of ethinylestradiol, norethindrone, and endogenous progesterone. *Obstet Gynecol* 1991;77:416–20

Orme ML'E, Back DJ. Interactions between oral contraceptive steroids and broad-spectrum antibiotics. *Clin Exp Dermatol* 1986;11:327–31

Swenson L, Goldin B, Gorbach SL. Effects of antibiotics on fecal/urinary excretion of ethinylestradiol, an oral contraceptive. *Gastroenterology* 1980;78:1332

3.9.3 COTRIMOXAZOLE

Documentation level	*Doubtful:* At least 17 pregnancies have been reported in the literature (Organon literature search, 1992). Whether these reported pregnancies should be attributed to a disturbance of the enterohepatic circulation of ethinylestradiol has not been investigated. In addition, the plasma concentrations of ethinylestradiol were significantly higher in women using cotrimoxazole concurrently as compared to controls (Grimmer *et al.*, 1983), making impairment of clinical efficacy unlikely.
Severity	*Minor:* The reported increase in plasma ethinylestradiol concentrations is of such a magnitude that no untoward effects are to be expected and therefore this interaction (if any) is of minor severity.
Mechanism of action	*Enzyme inhibition:* The inhibition probably concerns the inhibition of the oxidative metabolism since a similar interaction has been observed with cotrimoxazole and warfarin (O'Reilly, 1980) and it is thought that the sulfonamide component of cotrimoxazole is responsible for this action (Grimmer *et al.*, 1983).
Management	No evidence has been obtained indicating that clinically significant effects occur that would require adjustment of the dose or prescription of an alternative medication.
Clinically significant	No.

References	Grimmer SFM, Allen WL, Back DJ, *et al.* The effect of cotrimoxazole on oral contraceptive steroids in women. *Contraception* 1983;28:53–9
	O'Reilly RA. Stereoselective interaction of trimethoprim-sulfamethoxazole with the separated enantiomorphs of racemic warfarin in man. *N Engl J Med* 1980;302:33–5

3.9.4 DAPSONE

Documentation level	*Doubtful:* Although two pregnancies have been reported in the literature (Organon literature search, 1992), a pharmacokinetic study has shown that use of dapsone does not result in decreased plasma concentrations of norethisterone and ethinylestradiol. On the contrary, the plasma concentrations of ethinylestradiol were somewhat higher in women using dapsone concurrently as compared to controls (Joshi *et al.*, 1984).
Severity	*Minor:* The reported increase in plasma ethinylestradiol concentrations is of such a magnitude that no untoward effects are to be expected and therefore this interaction (if any) is of minor severity.
Mechanism of action	*Enzyme inhibition:* Mild enzyme inhibitory properties of dapsone have been reported previously in the guinea pig (Mier and Hurk, 1975). Further evidence for possible enzyme-inhibiting properties of dapsone comes from a study by Fleming *et al.* (1992) who suggested that dapsone bio trans-formation is mediated by cytochrome P_{450}IIIA4, the same enzyme system which is responsible for sex steroid metabolism.
Management	No evidence has been obtained indicating that clinically significant effects occur that would require adjustment of the dose or prescription of an alternative medication.
Clinically significant	No.

References	Fleming CM, Branch RA, Wilkinson GR, Guengerich FP. Human liver microsomal *N*-hydroxylation of dapsone by cytochrome P_{450}IIIA4. *Mol Pharmacol* 1992;41:975–80
	Joshi JV, Maitra A, Sankolli G, Bhatki S, Joshi UM. Norethisterone and ethinylestradiol kinetics during dapsone therapy. *J Assoc Phys India* 1984;32:191–3
	Mier PD, Hurk J. Inhibition of lysosomal enzymes by dapsone. *Br J Dermatol* 1975;93:471–2

3.9.5 GRISEOFULVIN

Documentation level	*Suspected:* There are four reported cases of unintended pregnancies (Organon literature search, 1992). In addition, there are a number of reports of cycle disturbances related to the concurrent use of oral contraceptives and griseofulvin (van Dijke and Weber, 1984). In one case, cycle irregularities disappeared after changing from a triphasic oral contraceptive to a monophasic 50 µg ethinylestradiol-containing oral contraceptive (McDaniel and Caldroney, 1986).
Severity	*Moderate:* This interaction is of moderate severity since the increased metabolism of contraceptive steroids may result in oral contraceptive failure.
Mechanism of action	*Enzyme induction:* Animal studies have shown that griseofulvin has enzyme-inducing properties (Denk *et al.*, 1977). In addition, griseofulvin interactions have also been reported with warfarin which were probably due to enzyme induction (Cullen and Catalano, 1967; Okino and Weibert, 1986).
Management	In the case of short-term concurrent drug treatment, a barrier method should be used both during concurrent drug treatment and for 7 days after discontinuation. If this would continue into the next oral contraceptive tablet-free interval, the woman should skip the tablet-free interval and start the next pack as soon as she has finished the pack in use.
Clinically significant	Yes.
References	Cullen SI, Catalano PM. Griseofulvin–warfarin antagonism. *J Am Med Assoc* 1967;199:582–3
	Denk H, Eckerstarfer R, Talcott RE, Schenkman JB. Alteration of hepatic microsomal enzymes by griseo-fulvin treatment of mice. *Biochem Pharmacol* 1977;26:1125–30

References

Dijke CPH van, Weber JCP. Interaction between oral contraceptives and griseofulvin. *Br Med J* 1984;288:1125–6

McDaniel PA, Caldroney RD. Oral contraceptives and griseofulvin interaction. *Drug Intell Clin Pharm* 1986;20:384

Okino K, Weibert RT. Warfarin–griseofulvin interaction. *Drug Intell Clin Pharm* 1986;20:291–2

3.9.6 RIFAMPICIN

Documentation level

Established: At least 27 pregnancies have been reported in the literature (Organon literature search, 1992). Further, several pharmacological and pharmacokinetic studies in women clearly show that rifampicin reduces oral contraceptive efficacy, as is apparent from increased follicular activity (Meyer *et al.*, 1987;1990) and decreased plasma concentrations of ethinylestradiol and norethisterone (Back *et al.*, 1979;1980a; Joshi *et al.*, 1980).

Severity

Moderate: This interaction is of moderate severity since the increased metabolism of contraceptive steroids may result in oral contraceptive failure.

Mechanism of action

Enzyme induction: There is convincing evidence that rifampicin induces a cytochrome P_{450} isoenzyme of the P_{450}IIIA subfamily (Combalbert *et al.*, 1989) which is also involved in the 2-hydroxylation of ethinylestradiol (Guengerich *et al.*, 1986; Guengerich, 1988). In addition, enzyme-inducing drugs are known to increase sex hormone binding globulin binding capacity (Victor *et al.*, 1977; Back *et al.*, 1980b).

Management

(1) In the case of short-term concurrent drug treatment, a barrier method should be used both during concurrent drug treatment and for 7 days after discontinuation. If this would continue into the next oral contraceptive tablet-free interval, the woman should skip the tablet-free interval and start the next pack as soon as she has finished the pack in use.

(2) In the case of long-term concurrent enzyme-inducing drug treatment:

– It is recommended to prescribe as a standard starting routine a monophasic 50 µg ethinylestradiol oral contraceptive (do not prescribe an oral contraceptive with placebo tablets, every-day pill).

– For example, the dosage regimen with this oral contraceptive could be four packs in a row followed by a tablet-free interval of 5 or 6 days.

– The contraceptive efficacy of the regimen can be judged on the basis of the occurrence of irregular bleeding (IB). IB is normally reviewed during the first follow-up visit (i.e. after the first four packs have been used). However, the woman should be advised that if IB is heavy and prolonged she should return sooner.

– If IB is too frequent:

- Increase the ethinylestradiol dose either by using a regimen of two sub-50 µg ethinylestradiol oral contraceptive tablets/day (i.e. 2 tablets with 30–35 µg ethinylestradiol/tablet) or a regimen of one 50 µg ethinylestradiol oral contraceptive tablet + one sub-50 µg ethinylestradiol oral contraceptive tablet/day.
- If IB still continues, increase the ethinylestradiol dose further to two 50 µg ethinylestradiol oral contraceptive tablets/day.
- If the above options are still not successful in controlling IB, the use of an alternative contraceptive method should be advised.

Note that after enzyme-inducing medication has been stopped, liver enzyme induction may be sustained during a period of approximately 4 weeks. Therefore, during this period, it is necessary either to stay on the higher dose oral contraceptive regimen or, when the woman resumes low-dose oral contraceptive use, in addition, to use a barrier method.

Clinically significant	Yes.

References	Back DJ, Breckenridge AM, Crawford F. The effect of rifampicin on norethisterone pharmacokinetics. *Eur J Clin Pharmacol* 1979;15:193–7
	Back DJ, Breckenridge AM, Crawford FE. The effect of rifampicin on the pharmacokinetics of ethinylestradiol in women. *Contraception* 1980a;21:135–43
	Back DJ, Breckenridge AM, Crawford FE, *et al*. The effect of oral contraceptive steroids and enzyme inducing drugs on sex hormone binding globulin capacity in women. *Br J Clin Pharmacol* 1980b; 9:115
	Combalbert J, Fabre I, Fabre G, *et al*. Metabolism of cyclosporin A. IV. Purification and identification of the rifampicin-inducible human liver cytochrome P_{450} (cyclosporin A oxidase) as a product of P_{450}IIIA gene subfamily. *Drug Metab Disp* 1989;17:197–207

References

Guengerich FP, Martin MV, Beaune PH, Kremers P, Wolff T, Waxman DJ. Characterization of rat and human liver microsomal cytochrome P_{450} forms involved in nifedipine oxidation, a prototype for genetic polymorphism in oxidative drug metabolism. *J Biol Chem* 1986;261:5051–60

Guengerich FP. Oxidation of 17α-ethinylestradiol by human liver cytochrome P_{450}. *Mol Pharmacol* 1988;33:500–8

Joshi JV, Joshi UM, Sankholi GM, *et al*. A study of interaction of a low-dose combination oral contraceptive with antitubercular drugs. *Contraception* 1980;21:617–29

Meyer BH, Müller FO, Luus H, Wessels P, Badian M, Röthig H-J. A model to investigate interactions obtunding oral contraceptive activity. *Med Sci Res* 1987;15:1497

Meyer B, Müller F, Wessels P, Maree J. A model to detect interactions between roxithromycin and oral contraceptives. *Clin Pharmacol Ther* 1990;47:671–4

Victor A, Lundberg PO, Johansson EDB. Induction of sex hormone binding globulin by phenytoin. *Br Med J* 1977; 2: 934–5

3.9.7 ISONIAZID

Documentation level	*Doubtful:* Although at least 14 pregnancies have been reported during use of isoniazid-containing multidrug therapy for tuberculosis (Organon literature search, 1992), these pregnancies must be attributed to rifampicin which was co-administered in all cases. This hypothesis is supported by a pharmacokinetic study that demonstrated unaltered plasma concentrations of both norethisterone and ethinylestradiol in women taking isoniazid-containing antituberculous drug therapy (Joshi *et al.*, 1980). In another study, it also appeared that isoniazid-containing therapy did not interfere with oral contraceptive efficacy (Mehrotra *et al.*, 1974).
Severity	*Not applicable:* There is probably no drug interaction between oral contraceptives and isoniazid.
Mechanism of action	*No mechanism:* There are no studies that point to a possible mechanism of interaction between this antimicrobial and oral contraceptives.
Management	No evidence has been obtained indicating that clinically significant effects occur that would require adjustment of the dose or prescription of an alternative medication.
Clinically significant	No.

References	Joshi JV, Joshi UM, Sankholi GM, *et al*. A study of interaction of a low-dose combination oral contraceptive with antitubercular drugs. *Contraception* 1980;21:617–29
	Mehrotra ML, Gautam KS, Pande DC, *et al*. Compatibility of oral contraceptive with antitubercular chemotherapy in female pulmonary tuberculosis patients. *India J Med Res* 1974;62:1782–6

3.9.8 TRIACETYLOLEANDOMYCIN

Documentation level	*Suspected:* At least 140 cases of hepatic cholestasis (exclusively from Belgium and France) resulting from a drug interaction between oral contraceptives and triacetyloleandomycin have been reported in the literature (Organon literature search, 1992).
Severity	*Moderate:* This interaction is of moderate severity since reversible hepatic damage may occur as a result of the concurrent use of oral contraceptives and triacetyloleandomycin.
Mechanism of action	*Enzyme inhibition:* Initially, triacetyloleandomycin induces cytochrome P_{450} isoenzymes (demethylases) that are responsible for the formation of nitrosalkane metabolites. These metabolites form stable inactive complexes with the iron center of cytochrome P_{450} enzymes. This leads subsequently to an inhibition of sex steroid metabolism, resulting in hepatic accumulation of these steroids with a direct toxic effect on the liver (Pessayre *et al.*, 1981; Fevery *et al.*, 1983). Other macrolides are not metabolized into nitrosalkanes and therefore are not expected to form inactive complexes with cytochrome P_{450} enzymes (Periti *et al.*, 1992).
Management	The concurrent use of oral contraceptives and triacetyloleandomycin should be avoided.
Clinically significant	Yes.

References	Fevery J, Steenbergen W van, Desmet V, *et al*. Severe intra-hepatic cholestasis due to the combined intake of oral contraceptives and triacetyloleandomycin. *Acta Clin Belg* 1983;38:242–5
	Periti P, Mazzei T, Mini E, Novelli A. Pharmacokinetic drug interactions of macrolides. *Clin Pharmacokinet* 1992;23:106–31
	Pessayre D, Konstantinova-Mitcheva M, Descatoire V, *et al*. Hypoactivity of cytochrome P_{450} after triacetyloleandomycin administration. *Biochem Pharmacol* 1981;30:559–64

3.9.9 OTHER ANTIMICROBIALS

Documentation level	*Doubtful:* Although some pregnancies have been reported with antimicrobial drugs such as metronidazole, cephalosporins, chloramphenicol, trimethoprim, erythromycin, sulfonamides and fusidic acid (Organon literature search, 1992), they have not been supported by pharmacological and/or pharmacokinetic interaction studies. Absence of drug interactions has been reported in studies using oral contraceptives concurrently with the macrolide antimicrobials, roxithromycin (Meyer *et al.*, 1990) and clarithromycin (Back *et al.*, 1991b), the imidazole antimycotics, ketoconazole (Back *et al.*, 1989) and fluconazole (Lazar and Wilner, 1990), the new imidazole derivative, SCH 39304 (Lunell *et al.*, 1991) and the quinoline derivative, temafloxacin (Back *et al.*, 1991a).
Severity	*Not applicable:* There are probably no drug interactions between oral contraceptives and the above-mentioned antimicrobial drugs.
Mechanism of action	*No mechanism:* There are no studies that point to a possible mechanism of interaction between these antimicrobials and oral contraceptives which could result in oral contraceptive failure.
Management	No evidence has been obtained indicating that clinically significant effects occur that would require adjustment of the dose or prescription of an alternative medication.
Clinically significant	No.

References	Back DJ, Stevenson P, Tjia JF. Comparative effects of two antimycotic agents, ketoconazole and terbinafine on the metabolism of tolbutamide, ethinylestradiol, cyclosporin and ethoxycoumarin by human liver microsomes *in vitro*. *Br J Clin Pharmacol* 1989;28:166–70
	Back DJ, Tjia J, Martin C, Millar E, Mant T, Morrison P, Orme M. The lack of interaction between temafloxacin and combined oral contraceptives. *Contraception* 1991a;43:317–23

References

Back DJ, Tjia J, Martin C, Millar E, Salmon P, Orme M. The interaction between clarithromycin and combined oral contraceptive steroids. *J Pharm Med* 1991b,2:81–7

Lazar JD, Wilner KD. Drug interactions with fluconazole. *Rev Infect Dis* 1990;12:S327–33

Lunell NO, Pschera H, Zador G, Carlström K. Evaluation of possible interaction of the antifungal triazole SCH 39304 with oral contraceptives in normal healthy women. *Gynecol Obstet Invest* 1991;32:91–7

Meyer B, Müller F, Wessels P, Maree J. A model to detect interactions between roxithromycin and oral contraceptives. *Clin Pharmacol Ther* 1990;47:671–4

3.10 ANTIPARASITICS

3.10a Effect of oral contraceptives on antiparasitic drug pharmacokinetics

Documentation level

Doubtful: From studies in monkeys (Dutta *et al.*, 1984) and in women (Karbwang *et al.*, 1988) infected with malaria, it appeared that the concurrent use of chloroquine and contraceptive steroids had no clinically significant effect on the efficacy of chloroquine. Pharmacokinetic drug interaction studies in women have shown that the pharmacokinetic parameters of chloroquine (Gupta *et al.*, 1984), mefloquine (Karbwang *et al.*, 1988), quinine (Wanwimolruk *et al.*, 1991) metronidazole (Joshi *et al.*, 1980) and mebendazole (Luder *et al.*, 1986) are not influenced by concurrent oral contraceptive use.

Severity

Not applicable: There is no evidence that antiparasitic drug pharmacokinetics are altered by concurrent oral contraceptive use.

Mechanism of action

No mechanism: There are no studies that point to a possible mechanism of action between antiparasitic drugs and oral contraceptives.

Management

No evidence has been obtained indicating that clinically significant effects occur that would require adjustment of the dose or prescription of an alternative medication.

Clinically significant

No.

3.10b Effect of antiparasitic drugs on oral contraceptive pharmacokinetics

Documentation level

Possible: Chloroquine has been shown to have no or only very weak enzyme-inhibiting properties on cytochrome P_{450}-dependent oxidative metabolic pathways (Back *et al.*, 1983a,b). Consequently, most experimental studies (Riviere and Back, 1986; Purba *et al.*, 1987) and clinical studies (Back *et al.*, 1984) have shown that chloroquine has no statistically significant effects on oral contraceptive pharmacokinetics. Quinoline derivatives, such as primaquine and mefloquine, have been shown to inhibit certain oxidative pathways (Back *et al.*, 1983b; Riviere and Back, 1985; Sukhumanan *et al.*, 1990). Although experimental studies have shown some inhibition of ethinylestradiol 2-hydroxylation by primaquine (Riviere and Back, 1985;1986; Purba *et al.*, 1987) and mefloquine, (Riviere and Back, 1986), a clinical study with primaquine indicated that oral contraceptive pharmacokinetics are not altered during concurrent drug treatment (Back et al., 1984). Thus, no evidence has been obtained that quinoline derivatives inhibit enzymes of the cytochrome $P_{450}IIIA$ subfamily, which is responsible for contraceptive steroid metabolism (Guengerich, 1990). Finally, it has also been shown that oral contraceptive pharmacokinetics are not altered by metronidazole (Joshi et al., 1980), praziquantel or metrifonate (El-Raghy et al., 1986).

Severity	**Minor**: Taking into account the reported magnitude of the above-mentioned changes in the metabolism of contraceptive steroids, the severity of this drug interaction is probably minor.
Mechanism of action	**Enzyme inhibition**: With some quinoline derivatives, inhibition of oral contraceptive-metabolizing enzymes has been suggested, but clinical studies did not reveal a clinically significant effect (Riviere and Back, 1985; 1986; Purba et al., 1987).
Management	No evidence has been obtained indicating that clinically significant effects occur that would require adjustment of the dose or prescription of an alternative medication.
Clinically significant	No.

References

Back DJ, Purba HS, Staiger C, Orme ML'E, Breckenridge AM. Inhibition of drug metabolism by the antimalarial drugs chloroquine and primaquine in the rat. *Biochem Pharmacol* 1983a;32:257–63

Back DJ, Purba HS, Park BK, Ward SA, Orme ML'E. Effect of chloroquine and primaquine on antipyrine metabolism. *Br J Clin Pharmacol* 1983b;16:497–502

Back DJ, Breckenridge AM, Grimmer SFM, Orme ML'E, Purba HS. Pharmacokinetics of oral contraceptive steroids following the administration of the antimalarial drugs primaquine and chloroquine. *Contraception* 1984;30:289–95

Dutta GP, Puri SK, Kamboj KK, Srivastava SK, Kamboj VP. Interactions between oral contraceptives and malaria infections in rhesus monkeys. *Bull WHO* 1984;62:931–9

References

El-Raghy I, Back DJ, Osman F, Orme ML'E, Fathalla M. Contraceptive steroid concentrations in women with early active schistosomiasis: lack of effect of antischistosomal drugs. *Contraception* 1986;33:373–7

Guengerich FP. Mechanism-based inactivation of human liver microsomal cytochrome $P_{450}IIIA4$ by gestodene. *Chem Res Toxicol* 1990;3:363–71

Gupta KC, Joshi JV, Desai NK *et al*. Kinetics of chloroquine and contraceptive steroids in oral contraceptive users during concurrent chloroquine prophylaxis. *India J Med Res* 1984;80:658–62

Joshi JV, Joshi VM, Sankholi GM *et al*. A study of interaction of low dose combination oral contraceptive with ampicillin and metronidazole[+]. *Contraception* 1980;22:643–52

Karbwang J, Looareesuwan S, Back DJ, Migasana S, Bunnag D, Breckenridge AM. Effect of oral contraceptive steroids on the clinical course of malaria infection and on the pharmacokinetics of mefloquine in Thai women. *Bull WHO* 1988;66:763–7

Luder PJ, Siffert B, Witassek F, Meister F, Bircher J. Treatment of hydatid disease with high oral doses of mebendazole. Long-term follow-up of plasma mebendazole levels and drug interactions. *Eur J Clin Pharmacol* 1986;31:443–8

Purba HS, Maggs JL, Orme ML'E, Back DJ, Park BK. The metabolism of 17α-ethinylestradiol by human liver microsomes: formation of catechol and chemically reactive metabolites. *Br J Clin Pharmacol* 1987;23:447–53

Riviere JH, Back DJ. Effect of mefloquine on hepatic drug metabolism in the rat: comparative study with primaquine. *Biochem Pharmacol* 1985;34:567–71

Riviere JH, Back DJ. Inhibition of ethinylestradiol and tolbutamide metabolism by quinoline derivatives *in vitro. Chem Biol Interact* 1986;59:301–8

Sukhumanan T, Suphakawanich W, Thithapandha A. Comparative inhibitory effects of mefloquine and primaquine on hepatic drug-metabolizing enzymes. *Biochem Pharmacol* 1990;39:212–16

Wanwimolruk S, Kaewvichit S, Tanthayaphinant O, Suwannarach C, Oranratnachai A. Lack of effect of oral contraceptive use on the pharmacokinetics of quinine. *Br J Clin Pharmacol* 1991;31:179–81

3.11 BENZODIAZEPINES

3.11.1 OXIDATIVELY METABOLIZED BENZODIAZEPINES

Documentation level	*Possible:* Although no clinical signs of altered benzodiazepine efficacy or increased incidence of benzodiazepine-related adverse reactions have been observed, a number of pharmacokinetic interaction studies (with high-dose oral contraceptives) have shown that the oxidative biotransformation of benzodiazepines is impaired, resulting in decreased total plasma clearance and an increased elimination half-life (Abernethy *et al.*, 1982; Patwardhan *et al.*, 1983). On the other hand, with low-dose oral contraceptives these changes in metabolism are less pronounced or even absent (Stoehr *et al.*, 1984; Ochs *et al.*, 1987; Scavone *et al.*, 1988).
Severity	*Minor:* Taking into account the reported magnitude of the above-mentioned changes in the metabolism of benzodiazepines and the large 'therapeutic window' of this class of drugs, the severity of this drug interaction is probably minor.
Mechanism of action	*Enzyme inhibition:* Both estrogens and progestagens are capable of inhibiting cytochrome $P_{450}IIIA$ activity in man (Back *et al.*, 1991; Chambers *et al.*, 1982; Guengerich, 1990). Since at least three benzodiazepines, diazepam, midazolam and triazolam, are oxidatively metabolized by cytochrome $P_{450}IIIA$ (Kronbach *et al.*, 1989; Reilly *et al.*, 1990), indirect evidence is provided for the mechanism of action resulting in impaired metabolism of certain benzodiazepines in oral contraceptive users.
Management	No evidence has been obtained indicating that clinically significant effects occur that would require adjustment of the dose or prescription of an alternative medication.
Clinically significant	No.
References	Abernethy DR, Greenblatt DJ, Divoll M, Arendt R. Impairment of diazepam clearance with low-dose oral contraceptive steroid therapy. *Clin Pharmacol Ther* 1982;31:198–9
	Back DJ, Houlgrave R, Tjia JF, Ward S, Orme ML'E. Effect of the progestogens, gestodene, 3-ketodesogestrel, levonorgestrel, norethisterone and norgestimate on the oxidation of ethinylestradiol and other substrates by human liver microsomes. *J Steroid Biochem Mol Biol* 1991;38:219–25

References

Chambers DM, Jefferson GC, Chambers M, Loudon NB. Antipyrine elimination in saliva after low-dose combined or progestogen-only contraceptive steroids. *Br J Clin Pharmacol* 1982;13:229–32

Guengerich FP. Mechanism-based inactivation of human liver microsomal cytochrome $P_{450}IIIA4$ by gestodene. *Chem Res Toxicol* 1990;3:363–71

Kronbach T, Mathys D, Umeno M, Gonzalez FJ, Meyer UA. Oxidation of midazolam and triazolam by human liver cytochrome $P_{450}IIIA4$. *Mol Pharmacol* 1989;36:89–96

Ochs HR, Greenblatt DJ, Friedman H, *et al*. Bromazepam pharmacokinetics: influence of age, gender, oral contraceptives, cimetidine, and propanolol. *Clin Pharmacol Ther* 1987;41:562–70

Patwardhan RV, Mitchell MC, Johnson RF, Schenker S. Differential effects of oral contraceptive steroids on the metabolism of benzodiazepines. *Hepatology* 1983;3:248–53

Reilly PEB, Thompson DA, Mason SR, Hooper WD. Cytochrome $P_{450}IIIA$ enzymes in rat liver microsomes: involvement in C3-hydroxylation of diazepam and nor-diazepam but not N-dealkylation of diazepam and temazepam. *Mol Pharmacol* 1990;37:767–74

Scavone JM, Greenblatt DJ, Locniskar A, Shader RI. Alprazolam pharmacokinetics in women on low-dose oral contraceptives. *J Clin Pharmacol* 1988;28:454–7

Stoehr GP, Kroboth PD, Juhl RP, *et al*. Effect of oral contraceptives on triazolam, temazepam, aprazolam and lorazepam kinetics. *Clin Pharmacol Ther* 1984;36:683–90

3.11.2 CONJUGATIVELY METABOLIZED BENZODIAZEPINES

Documentation level	*Possible:* Although no clinical signs of altered benzodiazepine efficacy or increased incidence of benzodiazepine-related adverse reactions have been reported, two pharmacokinetic interaction studies have shown that the conjugative biotransformation of benzodiazepines is accelerated, resulting in increased total plasma clearance and a decreased elimination half-life (Patwardhan *et al.*, 1983; Stoehr *et al.*, 1984). In a third study, however, no statistically significant changes in metabolism of such benzodiazepines have been observed (Abernethy *et al.*, 1983).
Severity	*Minor:* Taking into account the reported magnitude of the above-mentioned changes in the metabolism of benzodiazepines and the 'therapeutic window' of this class of drugs, the severity of this drug interaction is probably minor.
Mechanism of action	*Enzyme induction:* Although specific mechanism of action studies have not been performed, it is postulated that an enzyme-inducing effect of contraceptive steroids on hepatic uridine diphosphoglucuronosyltransferase activity is responsible for the enhanced conjugation of certain benzodiazepines (Patwardhan *et al.*, 1983; Miners *et al.*, 1984).
Management	No evidence has been obtained indicating that clinically significant effects occur that would require adjustment of the dose or prescription of an alternative medication.
Clinically significant	No.

References

Abernethy DR, Greenblatt DJ, Ochs HR, *et al.* Lorazepam and oxazepam kinetics in women on low-dose oral contraceptives. *Clin Pharmacol Ther* 1983;33:628–32

Miners JO, Deiner R, Attwood J, Robson R, Birkett DJ. Influence of sex and oral contraceptive steroids on drug glucuronidation. *Clin Exp Pharmacol Physiol* 1984; (Suppl 8):63

References

Patwardhan RV, Mitchell MC, Johnson RF, Schenker S. Differential effects of oral contraceptive steroids on the metabolism of benzodiazepines. *Hepatology* 1983;3:248–53

Stoehr GP, Kroboth PD, Juhl RP, *et al*. Effect of oral contraceptives on triazolam, temazepam, aprazolam and lorazepam kinetics. *Clin Pharmacol Ther* 1984;36:683–90

3.12 CORTICOSTEROIDS

Documentation level	*Possible:* Although *in vitro* data show a somewhat enhanced corticosteroid efficacy in oral contraceptive users (Frey and Frey, 1985), these effects have not been confirmed *in vivo*. In a number of studies, it has been shown that the biotransformation of prednisolone and cloprednol is impaired, resulting in a decreased total plasma clearance, an increased volume of distribution and an increased elimination half-life (Boekenoogen *et al.*, 1983; Frey *et al.*, 1984; Frey and Frey, 1985; Legler, 1987). In contrast, studies with fluocortolone show that its metabolism is not impaired in oral contraceptive users (Legler, 1988).
Severity	*Minor:* Taking into account the reported magnitude of the above- mentioned changes in the metabolism of corticosteroids and the large 'therapeutic window' of this class of drugs, the severity of this drug interaction is probably minor.
Mechanism of action	*Enzyme inhibition:* Both estrogens and progestagens are capable of inhibiting cytochrome $P_{450}IIIA$ activity in man (Chambers *et al.*, 1982; Back *et al.*, 1990; Guengerich, 1990). Since corticosteroids are also metabolized via the cytochrome P_{450} oxidative pathway (Boekenoogen *et al.*, 1983; Frey and Frey, 1983;1985; Gustavson *et al.*, 1986), there is indirect evidence that the mechanism of action is impaired metabolism of corticosteroids in oral contraceptive users. The reason why fluocortolone metabolism is not impaired in oral contraceptive users remains to be elucidated. An additional effect on free corticosteroid plasma levels resulting from oral contraceptive-induced changes in plasma corticosteroid binding globulin concentrations cannot be excluded (Boekenoogen *et al.*, 1983; Frey *et al.*, 1984; Gustavson and Benet, 1985).
Management	No evidence has been obtained indicating that clinically significant effects occur that would require adjustment of the dose or prescription of an alternative medication.
Clinically significant	No.

References

Back DJ, Houlgrave R, Tjia JF, Ward S, Orme ML'E. Effect of the progestogens, gestodene, 3-ketodesogestrel, levonorgestrel, norethisterone and norgestimate on the oxidation of ethinylestradiol and other substrates by human liver microsomes. *J Steroid Biochem Mol Biol* 1991;38:219–25

Boekenoogen SJ, Szefler SJ, Jasko WJ. Prednisolone disposition and protein binding in oral contraceptive users. *J Clin Endocrinol Metab* 1983;56:702–9

Chambers DM, Jefferson GC, Chambers M, Loudon NB. Antipyrine elimination in saliva after low-dose combined or progestogen-only contraceptive steroids. *Br J Clin Pharmacol* 1982;13:229–32

Frey FJ, Frey BM. Urinary 6β-hydroxyprednisolone excretion indicates enhanced prednisolone catabolism. *J Lab Clin Med* 1983;101:593–604

Frey BM, Schaad HJ, Frey FJ. Pharmacokinetic interaction of contraceptive steroids with prednisone and prednisolone. *Eur J Clin Pharmacol* 1984;26:505–11

Frey BM, Frey FJ. The effect of altered prednisolone kinetics in patients with the nephrotic syndrome and in women taking oral contraceptive steroids on human mixed lymphocyte cultures. *J Clin Endocrinol Metab* 1985;60:361–9

Guengerich FP. Mechanism-based inactivation of human liver microsomal cytochrome P_{450}IIIA4 by gestodene. *Chem Res Toxicol* 1990;3:363–71

Gustavson LE, Benet LZ. The macromolecular binding of prednisone in plasma of healthy volunteers including pregnant women and oral contraceptive users. *J Pharmacokinet Biopharm* 1985;13:561–9

Gustavson LE, Legler UF, Benet LZ. Impairment of prednisolone disposition in women taking oral contraceptives or conjugated estrogens. *J Clin Endocrinol Metab* 1986;62;234–7

Legler UF. Altered cloprednol disposition in oral contraceptive users. *Clin Pharmacol Ther* 1987;41:237

Legler UF. Lack of impairment of fluocortolone disposition in oral contraceptive users. *Eur J Clin Pharmacol* 1988;35:101–3

3.13 HYPOGLYCEMIC DRUGS

3.13a Effects of oral contraceptives on hypoglycemic drug pharmacokinetics

Documentation level	*Possible:* There are no clinical reports suggesting that the concurrent use of oral contraceptives and hypoglycemic drugs (either insulin or the oral hypoglycemic drugs such as tolbutamide) may lead to clinically significant drug interactions resulting in impaired antidiabetic drug biotransformation. In *in vitro* studies using human liver microsomes, ethinylestradiol (Purba *et al.*, 1987b) and various progestagens used in oral contraceptives (Back *et al.*, 1991) have been shown to be capable of inhibiting tolbutamide 4-hydroxylation. However, the clinical relevance of these findings is not clear.
Severity	*Minor:* Taking into account the magnitude of the above-mentioned changes in the metabolism of oral hypoglycemic drugs and the 'therapeutic window' of these drugs, the severity of this drug interaction is probably minor.
Mechanism of action	*Enzyme inhibition:* Because it is known that oral contraceptives inhibit hepatic mixed-function oxidases (Tephly and Mannering, 1968; Mackinnon *et al.*, 1977), it is theoretically possible that the metabolism of oral hypoglycemic drugs is impaired in oral contraceptive users. It has recently been found that two isoenzymes of the cytochrome $P_{450}IIC$ subfamily ($P_{450}IIC8$ and $P_{450}IIC9$) are responsible for tolbutamide 4-hydroxylation in man (Brian *et al.*, 1989; Relling *et al.*, 1990) and thus, it would be this isoenzyme which may be inhibited by contraceptive steroids.
Management	No evidence has been obtained indicating that clinically significant effects occur that would require adjustment of the dose or prescription of an alternative medication.
Clinically significant	No.

3.13b Effects of hypoglycemic drugs on oral contraceptive pharmacokinetics

Documentation level	*Doubtful:* There are no clinical reports suggesting that the concurrent use of oral contraceptives and hypoglycemic drugs (either insulin or the oral hypoglycemic drugs such as tolbutamide) may lead to clinically significant drug interactions resulting in inhibition of oral contraceptive biotransformation. However, an experimental *in vitro* study using human liver microsomes showed that tolbutamide may, to some extent, inhibit ethinylestradiol 2-hydroxylation (Purba *et al.*, 1987a).
Severity	*Minor:* Taking into account the reported magnitude of the above-mentioned changes in the metabolism of ethinylestradiol, the clinical relevance of *in vitro* findings (for example, inhibition of ethinylestradiol 2-hydroxylation may be compensated for by increased sulfation and conjugation), the severity of this drug interaction (if any) is probably minor.
Mechanisms of action	*Enzyme inhibition:* Cytochrome $P_{450}IIIA4$ has been identified as the major ethinylestradiol-metabolizing enzyme (Guengerich, 1988). This isoenzyme may be inhibited by tolbutamide (Purba *et al.*, 1987a)
Management	No evidence has been obtained indicating that clinically significant effects occur that would require adjustment of the dose or prescription of an alternative medication.
Clinically significant	No.

References	Back DJ, Houlgrave R, Tjia JF, Ward S, Orme ML'E. Effect of the progestogens, gestodene, 3-ketodesogestrel, levonorgestrel, norethisterone and norgestimate on the oxidation of ethinylestradiol and other substrates by human liver microsomes. *J Steroid Biochem Mol Biol* 1991;38:219–25
	Brian WR, Srivastava PK, Umbenhauer DR, Lloyd RS, Guengerich FP. Expression of a human liver cytochrome P_{450} protein with tolbutamide hydroxylase activity in *Saccharomyces cereviciae. Biochemistry* 1989;28:4993–9
	Guengerich FP. Oxidation of 17α-ethinylestradiol by human liver cytochrome P_{450}. *Mol Pharmacol* 1988;33:500–8

References

Mackinnon M, Sutherland E, Simon FE. Effects of ethinyl-estradiol on hepatic microsomal proteins and the turnover of cytochrome P_{450}. *J Lab Clin Med* 1977;90:1096–106

Purba HS, Maggs JL, Orme ML'E, Back DJ, Park BK. The metabolism of 17α-ethinylestradiol by human liver microsomes: formation of catechol and chemically reactive metabolites. *Br J Clin Pharmacol* 1987a;23:447–53

Purba HS, Back DJ, Orme ML'E. Tolbutamide 4-hydroxylase activity of human liver microsomes: effect of inhibitors. *Br J Clin Pharmacol* 1987b;24:230–4

Relling MV, Aoyama T, Gonzalez FJ, Meyer UA. Tolbutamide and mephenytoin hydroxylation by human cytochrome P_{450} in the CYP2C subfamily. *J Pharmacol Exp Ther* 1990;252:442–7

Tephly TR, Mannering GJ. Inhibition of drug metabolism. *Mol Pharmacol* 1968;4:10–14

3.14 IMMUNOSUPPRESSANTS

Documentation level	*Possible:* A number of case reports have appeared associating the concurrent use of combined oral contraceptives (Leimenstoll *et al.*, 1984; Deray *et al.*, 1987) or other synthetic sex hormones (Möller and Ekelund, 1985; Ross *et al.*, 1986; Jonon *et al.*, 1989) and the immunosuppressant drug, cyclosporin, with hepatotoxicity. The liver disturbances appeared to be reversible, as on discontinuation of sex hormone treatment, cholestasis improved, which was measured by disappearance of clinical symptoms and the rapid decline of pathologically increased hepatic laboratory parameters. The interaction between sex hormones and cyclosporin has, however, not been substantiated in well-designed clinical studies.
Severity	*Moderate:* The interaction is of moderate severity since reversible hepatic damage may occur as a result of the concurrent use of oral contraceptives and cyclosporin.
Mechanism of action	*Enzyme inhibition:* From biochemical studies, evidence has been obtained that cyclosporin is metabolized mainly via cytochrome $P_{450}IIIA$ (Kronbach *et al.*, 1988; Watkins, 1990). Cytochrome $P_{450}IIIA$ is also responsible for metabolism of contraceptive steroids in man (Chambers *et al.*, 1982; Guengerich, 1990; Back *et al.*, 1991). Consequently, as the cytochrome $P_{450}IIIA$ pool appears to be a rate-limiting factor in the metabolism of both cyclosporin and sex hormones (Watkins, 1990), competitive inhibition of either cyclosporin or sex steroid metabolism (or both) cannot be excluded. From three recent *in vitro* studies using human hepatocytes and/or liver microsomes, it appeared that in these test systems estradiol (Henricsson *et al.*, 1990) ethinylestradiol, progesterone (Pichard *et al.*, 1990) and synthetic progestagens (Back *et al.*, 1991) were all competitive inhibitors of cyclosporin metabolism. Surprisingly, in an *in vitro* study in perfused rat liver, the metabolism of cyclosporin appeared to be increased in ethinylestradiol-treated rats as compared to controls (Prueksaritanont *et al.*, 1992).
Management	No evidence has been obtained indicating that clinically significant effects occur that would require adjustment of the dose or prescription of an alternative medication.
Clinically significant	No.

References

Back DJ, Houlgrave R, Tjia JF, Ward S, Orme ML'E. Effect of the progestogens, gestodene, 3-ketodesogestrel, levonorgestrel, norethisterone and norgestimate on the oxidation of ethinylestradiol and other substrates by human liver microsomes. *J Steroid Biochem Mol Biol* 1991;38:219–25

Chambers DM, Jefferson GC, Chambers M, Loudon NB. Antipyrine elimination in saliva after low-dose combined or progestogen-only contraceptive steroids. *Br J Clin Pharmacol* 1982;13:229–32

Deray G, Hoang P le, Cacoub P, Assogba U, Grippon P, Baumelou A. Oral contraceptive interaction with cyclosporin. *Lancet* 1987;1:158–9

Guengerich FP. Mechanism-based inactivation of human liver microsomal cytochrome $P_{450}IIIA4$ by gestodene. *Chem Res Toxicol* 1990;3:363–71

Henricsson S, Lindholm A, Aravoglou M. Cyclosporin metabolism in human liver microsome and its inhibition by other drugs. *Pharmacol Toxicol* 1990;66:49–52

Jonon B, Lataste A, Renoult E, Kessler M. Problèmes posés par l'utilisation des progestatifs chez la femme transplantée rénale traitée par ciclosporine. *Ann Med Nancy Est* 1989;28:183–6

Kronbach T, Fischer V, Meyer UA. Cyclosporin metabolism in human liver: identification of a cytochrome $P_{450}III$ gene family as the major cyclosporin-metabolizing enzyme explains interactions of cyclosporin with other drugs. *Clin Pharmacol Ther* 1988;43:630–5

Leimenstoll G, Jessen P, Zabel P, Niedermayer W. Arzneimittelschädigung der Leber bei Kombination von Cyclosporin A und einem antikonzeptivum. *Dtsch Med Wochenschr* 1984;109:1989–90

Möller BB, Ekelund B. Toxicity of cyclosporin during treatment with androgens. *N Engl J Med* 1985;313:1416

Pichard L, Fabre I, Fabre G, Domergue J, Saint Aubert B, Mourad G, *et al*. Cyclosporin A drug interaction. *Drug Metab Dispos* 1990;18:595–606

References

Prueksaritanont T, Hoener BA, Benet LZ. Effects of low-density lipoproteins and ethinylestradiol on cyclosporin metabolism in isolated rat liver perfusions. *Drug Metab Disp* 1992;20:547–52

Ross WB, Roberts D, Griffin PJA, Salaman JR. Cyclosporin interaction with danazol and norethisterone. *Lancet* 1986;1:330

Watkins PB. The role of cytochromes P_{450} in cyclosporin metabolism. *J Am Acad Dermatol* 1990;23:1301–11

3.15 LAXATIVES

Documentation level	*Doubtful:* There is only one case report on a pregnancy attributed to an interaction between oral contraceptives and laxatives (Köhler *et al.*, 1976). Pharmacodynamic and pharmacokinetic data are lacking.
Severity	*Moderate:* This interaction is of moderate severity since decreased absorption of contraceptive steroids may result in oral contraceptive failure.
Mechanism of action	*Decreased absorption:* Theoretically, only those laxatives which produce a watery evacuation within 3 hours of administration (these types of very strong and fast-working laxatives are also called cathartics) may be capable of reducing the efficacy of oral contraceptives. This is because contraceptive steroids are absorbed rapidly and completely (Orme *et al.*, 1983). Therefore, only saline cathartics (which act by water retention in the bowel) and castor oil and liquid paraffin (which might interfere with the absorption of fat-soluble substances) could theoretically induce a disturbed absorption of contraceptive steroids (Swyer, 1969; Husmann, 1978; Brunton, 1990). However, relevant clinical data are not available. In addition, laxatives which act primarily on the colon (bulk formers, bisacodyl and related compounds, anthraquinones) are not expected to interact with oral contraceptives, since the latter are absorbed from the upper part of the small intestine (Zielske, 1982; Svensson, 1985).
Management	No evidence has been obtained indicating that clinically significant effects occur that would require adjustment of the dose or prescription of an alternative medication.
Clinically significant	No.
References	Brunton LL. Agents affecting gastrointestinal water flux and motility, digestants and bile acids. In: Goodman-Gilman A, Rall Th W, Nies AS, Taylor P, eds. *The Pharmacological Basis of Therapeutics*, 8th edn. New York: Pergamon Press, 1990;914–32

References

Husmann F. Arzneimittelinteraktionen unter der Behandlung mit hormonalen Kontrazeptiva. *Therapiewoche* 1978;28:9352–6

Köhler E, Stein W, Mohr U. Gemeinschaftsuntersuchung über die Wirksamkeit und Zykluskontrolle eines modifizierten oralen Sequenzkontrazeptivums. *Prakt Arzt* 1976;30:943–51

Orme M, Back DJ, Breckenridge AM. Clinical pharmacology of oral contraceptive steroids. *Clin Pharmacokinet* 1983;8:95–136

Svensson WE. Bowel preparation and the pill. *Clin Radiol* 1985;36:340

Swyer GIM. Liquid paraffin and oral contraception. *Practitioner* 1969;202:592

Zielske F. Laxantien und hormonale Kontrazeptiva. *Dtsch Med Wochenschr* 1982;107:1650–1

3.16 METHYLXANTHINES

3.16.1 THEOPHYLLINE

Documentation level	*Possible:* Most studies have shown that the metabolism of theophylline is impaired in women using oral contraceptives as compared to controls, as measured by decreased plasma clearance and an increased elimination half-life (Jusko *et al.*, 1979; Tornatore *et al.*, 1982; Gardner *et al.*, 1983; Roberts *et al.*, 1983). However, the observed inhibition of plasma clearance is below the level needed to induce clinically relevant adverse drug experiences (Schentag, 1993). On the other hand, a recent study did not show inhibition of theophylline metabolism in oral contraceptive users (Koren *et al.*, 1985). This can be attributed to the finding that enzyme inhibition only takes place during the initial period of concurrent drug treatment and subsequently tends to normalize with time. Evidence for this latter explanation has recently accumulated from long-term drug interaction studies with caffeine (which is pharmacologically similar to theophylline) and oral contraceptives (Balogh *et al.*, 1991).
Severity	*Minor:* Taking into account the reported magnitude of the above-mentioned changes in the metabolism of theophylline and the 'therapeutic window' of this class of drugs, the severity of this drug interaction is probably minor.
Mechanism of action	*Enzyme inhibition:* Both estrogens and progestagens are capable of inhibiting cytochrome P_{450} activity in man (Chambers *et al.*, 1982; Back *et al.*, 1990; Guengerich, 1990) and indeed it was found that the greatest inhibition of theophylline metabolism occurred in subjects with the highest area under curves for both norgestrel and ethinylestradiol (Gardner *et al.*, 1983). Theophylline is metabolized via various cytochrome P_{450}-dependent metabolic pathways, with cytochrome $P_{450}IA2$ probably playing a major role in *N*-demethylation of theophylline (Ratanasavananh *et al.*, 1990) and another isoenzyme being responsible for 8-hydroxylation. In oral contraceptive users, *N*-demethylation of theophylline is impaired to a greater extent as compared to the other routes of metabolism (Gardner and Jusko, 1986; Sarkar *et al.*, 1990).
Management	No evidence has been obtained indicating that clinically significant effects occur that would require adjustment of the dose or prescription of an alternative medication.
Clinically significant	No.

References

Back DJ, Houlgrave R, Tjia JF, Ward S, Orme HL'E. Effect of the progestogens, gestodene, 3-ketodesogestrel, levonorgestrel, norethisterone and norgestimate on the oxidation of ethinylestradiol and other substrates by human liver microsomes. *J Steroid Biochem Mol Biol* 1991;38:219–25

Balogh A, Irmisch E, Wolf P, Letrari S, Splinter FK, Hempel E, *et al*. Zum Einfluß von Levonorgestrel und Ethinylestradiol sowie deren Kombination auf die Aktivität von Biotransformationsreaktionen. *Zentralbl Gynaekol* 1991;113:1388–96

Chambers DM, Jefferson GC, Chambers M, Loudon NB. Antipyrine elimination in saliva after low-dose combined or progestogen-only contraceptive steroids. *Br J Clin Pharmacol* 1982;13:229–32

Gardner MJ, Tornatore KM, Jusko WJ, Kanarkowski R. Effects of tobacco smoking and oral contraceptive use on theophylline disposition. *Br J Clin Pharmacol* 1983;16:271–80

Gardner MJ, Jusko WJ. Effects of oral contraceptives and tobacco use on the metabolic pathways of theophylline. *Int J Pharmaceut* 1986;33:55–64

Guengerich FP. Mechanism-based inactivation of human liver microsomal cytochrome P_{450}IIIA4 by gestodene. *Chem Res Toxicol* 1990;3:363-71

Jusko WJ, Gardner MJ, Mangione A, Schentag JJ, Koup JR, Vance JW. Factors affecting theophylline clearances: age, tobacco, marijuana, cirrhosis, congestive heart failure, obesity, oral contraceptives, benzodiazepines, barbiturates, and ethanol. *J Pharm Sci* 1979;68:1358–66

Koren G, Chin TF, Correia J, Tesoro A, MacLeod SM. Theophylline pharmacokinetics in adolescent females following coadministration of oral contraceptives. *Clin Invest Med* 1985;8:222–6

Ratanasavananh D, Berthou F, Dreano Y, Mondine P, Guillouzo A, Riche C. Methylcholantrene but not phenobarbital enhances caffeine and theophylline metabolism in cultured adult human hepatocytes. *Biochem Pharmacol* 1990;39:85–94

References

Roberts RK, Grice J, McGuffie C, Heilbronn L. Oral contraceptive steroids impair elimination of theophylline. *J Lab Clin Med* 1983;101:821–5

Sarkar M, Polk RE, Guzelian PS, Hunt C, Karnes HT. *In vitro* effect of fluoroquinolones on theophylline metabolism in human liver microsomes. *Antimicrob Agents Chemother* 1990;34:594–9

Schentag JJ. Assessment of pharmacokinetic drug interactions in clinical drug development. In: Yacobi A, Skelly JP, Shah VP, Benet LZ, eds. *Integration of Pharmacokinetics, Pharmacodynamics, and Toxicokinetics in Rational Drug Development.* New York: Plenum Press, 1993: 149–57

Tornatore KM, Kanarkowski R, McCarthy TL, Gardner MJ, Yurchak AM, Jusko WJ. Effect of chronic oral contraceptive steroids on theophylline disposition. *Eur J Clin Pharmacol* 1982;23:129–34

3.16.2 CAFFEINE

Documentation level

Possible: Similar to the interaction studies between oral contraceptives and theophylline, also the metabolism of caffeine has been reported to be impaired by concurrent use of oral contraceptives. In general, it was found that caffeine plasma clearance is decreased and that the elimination half-life is increased in oral contraceptive users (Patwardhan *et al.*, 1980; Rietveld *et al.*, 1984; Abernethy and Todd, 1985; Campbell *et al.*, 1987; Bergmann *et al.*, 1988; Meyer *et al.*, 1988). In recent studies, however, it appeared that significant enzyme inhibition occurred only during short-term concurrent use of oral contraceptives and caffeine, but that after long-term use all parameters had returned to baseline values despite continuation of treatment with both oral contraceptives and caffeine (Meyer *et al.*, 1989; Balogh *et al.*, 1991). This suggests that enzyme inhibition takes place only during the initial period of concurrent drug treatment and subsequently tends to normalize with time.

Further, it has been reported that caffeine metabolism is impaired to a greater extent in moderately hypertensive oral contraceptive users as compared to normotensive oral contraceptive users, which has been attributed to the higher ethinylestradiol plasma levels in women with high blood pressure (Kaul and Ahluwalia, 1988).

Severity

Minor: Taking into account the reported magnitude of the above-mentioned changes in the metabolism of caffeine and the 'therapeutic window' of this class of drugs, the severity of this drug interaction is probably minor.

Mechanism of action

Enzyme inhibition: Both estrogens and progestagens are capable of inhibiting cytochrome P_{450} activity in man (Chambers *et al.*, 1982; Guengerich, 1990; Back *et al.*, 1991). Caffeine is metabolized by at least two isoenzymes of the cytochrome P_{450} system with cytochrome $P_{450}IA2$ being the major isoenzyme responsible for the N-demethylation and another isoenzyme being responsible for the 8-hydroxylation, similar to the theophylline metabolic pathway (Grant *et al.*, 1987; Ratanasavananh *et al.*, 1990). It has indeed been shown that caffeine N-demethylation by cytochrome $P_{450}IA2$ in oral contraceptive users is impaired to a greater extent as compared to the other routes of caffeine metabolism (Campbell *et al.*, 1987; Kalow and Tang, 1991).

Management	No evidence has been obtained indicating that clinically significant effects occur that would require adjustment of the dose or prescription of an alternative medication.
Clinically significant	No.

References

Abernethy DR, Todd EL. Impairment of caffeine clearance by chronic use of low-dose estrogen-containing oral contraceptives. *Eur J Clin Pharmacol* 1985;28:425–8

Back DJ, Houlgrave R, Tjia JF, Ward S, Orme ML'E. Effect of the progestogens, gestodene, 3-ketodesogestrel, levonorgestrel, norethisterone and norgestimate on the oxidation of ethinylestradiol and other substrates by human liver microsomes. *J Steroid Biochem Mol Biol* 1991;38:219–25

Balogh A, Irmisch E, Wolf P, Letrari S, Splinter FK, Hempel E, *et al.* Zum Einfluβ von Levonorgestrel und Ethinylestradiol sowie deren Kombination auf die Aktivität von Biotransformationsreaktionen. *Zentralbl Gynaekol* 1991;113:1388–96

Bergmann M, Splinter FC, Henschel L, Balogh A, Hoffmann A, Klinger G. Die Metamizol-Coffein-Elimination bei Frauen mit erhöhten Aminotransferase-Aktivitäten im Serum unter steroidalen oralen Kontrazeptiva. *Dtsch Z Verdau Stoffwechselkrankh* 1988;48:261–7

Campbell ME, Spielberg SP, Kalow W. A urinary metabolite ratio that reflects systemic caffeine clearance. *Clin Pharmacol Ther* 1987;42:157–65

Chambers DM, Jefferson GC, Chambers M, Loudon NB. Antipyrine elimination in saliva after low-dose combined or progestogen-only contraceptive steroids. *Br J Clin Pharmacol* 1982;13:229–32

Grant DM, Campbell ME, Tang BK, Kalow W. Biotransformation of caffeine by microsomes from human liver. *Biochem Pharmacol* 1987;36:1251–60

Guengerich FP. Mechanism-based inactivation of human liver microsomal cytochrome P_{450}IIIA4 by gestodene. *Chem Res Toxicol* 1990;3:363–71

References

Kalow W, Tang BK. Use of caffeine metabolite ratios to explore CYPIA2 and xanthine oxidase activities. *Clin Pharmacol Ther* 1991;50:508–19

Kaul L, Ahluwalia B. Inter-relation of caffeine and oral contraceptive OC steroid metabolism in hypertensive OC users in humans. *J Steroid Biochem* 1988;37:1651–9

Meyer FP, Canzler E, Giers H, Walther H. Langzeituntersuchung zum Einfluss von Non-Ovlon auf die Pharmakokinetic von Coffein im intraindividuellen Vergleich. *Zentralbl Gynaekol* 1988;110:1449–54

Meyer FP, Walther H, Canzler E, Giers H. Einfluss der oralen Kontrazeptiva Minisiston/Trisiston auf die Pharmakokinetic von Coffein–ein intraindividueller Langzeitvergleich. *Z Klin Med* 1989;44:239–40

Patwardhan RV, Desmond PV, Johnson RF, Schenker SS. Impaired elimination of caffeine by oral contraceptive steroids. *J Lab Clin Med* 1980;95:603–8

Ratanasavananh D, Berthou F, Dreano Y, Mondine P, Guillouzo A, Riche C. Methylcholantrene but not phenobarbital enhances caffeine and theophylline metabolism in cultured adult human hepatocytes. *Biochem Pharmacol* 1990;39:85–94

Rietveld EC, Broekman MMM, Houben JJG, Eskes TKAB, Rossum JM van. Rapid onset of an increase in caffeine residence time in young women due to oral contraceptive use. *Eur J Clin Pharmacol* 1984;26:371–3

3.17 SMOKING

Documentation level	*Possible:* One study reported an increased incidence of oral contraceptive failure in smokers (Sparrow, 1989), whereas another did not (Vessey *et al.*, 1987). A causative relationship could not be established. Also, clinical pharmacological studies show contradictory results: Crawford *et al.* (1981) found no induction of biotransformation of levonorgestrel or ethinylestradiol, whereas in another study, indications of enzyme induction of ethinylestradiol were found (Kanarkowski *et al.*, 1988).
Severity	*Moderate:* This interaction is of moderate severity since the increased metabolism of contraceptive steroids may result in oral contraceptive failure.
Mechanism of action	*Enzyme induction:* In humans, cigarette smoking increases the cytochrome P_{450}-dependent oxidative metabolism of estradiol (Michnovicz *et al.*, 1986). This effect is of clinical importance because cigarette smoking has, due to this induction of estradiol biotransformation, an antiestrogenic effect. Estradiol is oxidized usually either to estrone, which is metabolized further to 16α-hydroxyestrone and subsequently to estriol, or to 2-hydroxyestrone and subsequently to 2-methoxyestrone. The metabolites formed by 2-hydroxylation are virtually devoid of estrogenic activity, whereas those formed by 16α-hydroxylation have potent estrogenic activity (Miller, 1990; Shulman *et al.*, 1990). Cigarette smoking exerts its antiestrogenic activity especially by inducing the 2-hydroxylation pathway of estradiol (Michnovicz *et al.*, 1986).
	Biochemical indications for absence of a drug interaction between smoking and ethinylestradiol (but not between smoking and estradiol) came from an *in vitro* study using human liver microsomes. It appeared from this study that 2-hydroxylation of estradiol is catalyzed by enzymes of the cytochrome $P_{450}IA$ family, whereas the 2-hydroxylation of ethinylestradiol in man is catalyzed by cytochromes of other genes (i.e. $P_{450}IIC$, $P_{450}IIE$ and $P_{450}IIIA$), thus differentiating between estradiol and ethinylestradiol 2-hydroxylation (Ball *et al.*, 1990).
Management	No evidence has been obtained indicating that clinically significant effects occur that would require adjustment of the dose or prescription of an alternative medication.
Clinically significant	No.

References

Ball SE, Forrester LM, Wolf CR, Back DJ. Differences in the cytochrome P_{450} isozymes involved in the 2-hydroxylation of estradiol and 17α-ethinylestradiol: relative activities of rat and human liver enzymes. *Biochem J* 1990;267:221–6

Crawford FE. Back DJ, Orme ML'E, Breckenridge AM. Oral contraceptive steroid plasma concentrations in smokers and non-smokers. *Br Med J* 1981;282:1829–30

Kanarkowski R, Tornatore KM, D'Ambrosio R, Gardner MJ, Jusko WJ. Pharmacokinetics of single and multiple doses of ethinylestradiol and levonorgestrel in relation to smoking. *Clin Pharmacol Ther* 1988;43:23–31

Michnovicz JJ, Hershcopf RJ, Naganuma H, Bradlow HL, Fishman J. Increased 2-hydroxylation of estradiol as a possible mechanism for the anti-estrogenic effect of cigarette smoking. *N Engl J Med* 1986;315:1305–9

Miller LG. Cigarettes and drug therapy: pharmacokinetic and pharmacodynamic considerations. *Clin Pharm* 1990;9:125–35

Shulman A, Ellenbogen A, Maymon R, Bahary C. Smoking out the estrogens. *Hum Reprod* 1990;5:231–3

Sparrow MJ. Pregnancies in reliable pill takers. *NZ Med J* 1989;102:575–7

Vessey MP, Villard-Mackintosh L, Jacobs HS. Anti-estrogenic effect of cigarette smoking. *N Engl J Med* 1987;317:769–70

3.18 VITAMINS

3.18.1 VITAMIN A AND DERIVATIVES

3.18.1a Effect of oral contraceptives on vitamin A pharmacokinetics

Documentation level	*Doubtful:* No cases of oral contraceptive-induced hypovitaminosis A have been reported. In a World Health Organization study, it was reported that oral contraceptive use did not worsen existing vitamin A malnutrition (Joshi *et al.*, 1986). Animal data have indicated that absorption and excretion of vitamin A are not impaired by use of contraceptive steroids (Supopark and Olson, 1975). In fact, human studies unanimously have reported increased plasma levels of vitamin A in oral contraceptive users as compared to controls (Gal *et al.*, 1971; Yeung, 1976; Palan *et al.*, 1989; Mooij *et al.*, 1991). The increased vitamin A plasma levels in oral contraceptive users remained far below toxic and/or teratogenic levels (Mooij *et al.*, 1991). This has been confirmed by the absence of fetal malformations in the offspring of women with high oral contraceptive-induced vitamin A plasma levels prior to pregnancy (Wild *et al.*, 1974).
Severity	*Major:* If vitamin A levels were to be increased to teratogenic levels, this could result in serious adverse reactions in the offspring of previous oral contraceptive users.
Mechanism of action	*Protein binding:* The early studies suggested that there may be an increased metabolism of provitamin A to vitamin A (Gal *et al.*, 1971; Horwitt *et al.*, 1975), but most authors nowadays consider the increased plasma concentrations of vitamin A, as found in oral contraceptive users, to be due to the increased plasma concentration of the carrier protein of vitamin A – retinol-binding protein (Vahlquist *et al.*, 1979; Nonavinakere *et al.*, 1981; Mooij *et al.*, 1991). The increase appeared to be estrogen dose-dependent as was shown by controlled studies (Horwitt *et al.*, 1975).
Management	No evidence has been obtained indicating that clinically significant effects occur that would require adjustment of the dose or prescription of an alternative medication.
Clinically significant	No.

3.18.1b Effect of vitamin A derivatives on oral contraceptive pharmacokinetics

Documentation level	*Doubtful:* In a study using the synthetic vitamin A derivative, isotretinoin, and oral contraceptives concurrently, it appeared that isotretinoin had no influence on plasma concentrations of both levonorgestrel and ethinylestradiol (Orme *et al.*, 1984). In another study, the concurrent use of oral contraceptives and acitretin did not interfere with oral contraceptive efficacy, as measured by plasma progesterone levels before, during and after the trial (Berbis *et al.*, 1988).
Severity	*Major:* If synthetic vitamin A derivatives were able to reduce oral contraceptive efficacy and if an oral contraceptive user were to become accidentally pregnant, the fetus would be exposed to high levels of these substances which may result in teratogenic effects.
Mechanism of action	*No mechanism:* Synthetic vitamin A derivatives do not appear to have enzyme-inducing properties.
Management	No evidence has been obtained indicating that clinically significant effects occur that would require adjustment of the dose or prescription of an alternative medication.
Clinically significant	No.

References

Berbis P, Bun H, Geiger JM, Rognin C, Durand A, Serradimigni A, *et al.* Acitretin (R010-1670) and oral contraceptives: interaction study. *Arch Dermatol Res* 1988;280:388–9

Gal I, Parkinson C, Craft I. Effects of oral contraceptives on human plasma vitamin A levels. *Br Med J* 1971;2:436–8

Horwitt MK, Harvey CC, Dahm CH. Relationship between levels of blood lipids, vitamins C, A and E, serum copper compounds, and urinary excretions of tryptophan metabolites in women taking oral contraceptive therapy. *Am J Clin Nutr* 1975;28:403–12

References

Joshi UM, Virkar KD, Amatayakul K, Singkamani R, Bamji MS, Prema K, *et al.* Impact of hormonal contraceptives vis-a-vis non-hormonal factors on the vitamin status of malnourished women in India and Thailand. *Hum Nutr Clin Nutr* 1986;40C:205–20

Mooij PNM, Thomas CMG, Doesburg WH, Eskes TKAB. Multivitamin supplementation in oral contraceptive users. *Contraception* 1991;44:277–88

Nonavinakere VK, Man YM, Lei KY. Oral contraceptives, norethindrone and mestranol: effect on serum vitamin A, retinol-binding protein and prealbumin levels in women. *Nutr Rep Int* 1981;23:697–704

Orme M, Back DJ, Cunliffe WJ, Jones DH, Allen WL, Tjia J. Isotretinoin and oral contraceptive steroids. *Br J Clin Pharmacol* 1984;17:227P–228P

Palan PR, Romney SL, Vermund SH, Mikhail MG, Basu J. Effects of smoking and oral contraceptives on plasma β-carotene levels in healthy women. *Am J Obstet Gynecol* 1989;161:881–5

Supopark W, Olson JA. Effect of Ovral, a combination type oral contraceptive agent, on vitamin A metabolism in rats. *Int J Vitam Nutr Res* 1975;45:113–23

Vahlquist A, Johnsson A, Nygren KG. Vitamin A transporting plasma proteins and female sex hormones. *Am J Clin Nutr* 1979;32:1433–8

Wild J, Schorah CJ, Smithells RW. Vitamin A, pregnancy and oral contraceptives. *Br Med J* 1974;1:57–9

Yeung DL. Relationship between cigarette smoking, oral contraceptives, and plasma vitamins A, E, C, and plasma triglycerides and cholesterol. *Am J Clin Nutr* 1976;29:1216–21

3.18.2 VITAMIN B₁ (THIAMINE)

Documentation level	*Doubtful:* From various studies it appeared that oral contraceptive use did not influence adversely vitamin B_1 status in either vitamin B_1-supplemented (Lewis and King, 1980) or non-supplemented healthy women (Ahmed *et al.*, 1975; Vir and Love, 1979). In a multicenter World Health Organization study, however, it appeared that there was a slight improvement in vitamin B_1 status in non-supplemented under-nourished Indian oral contraceptive users as compared to baseline, whereas there was a small deterioration in vitamin B_1 status in non-supplemented well-nourished Thai oral contraceptive users. These small biochemical changes were not considered clinically relevant (Joshi *et al.*, 1986).
Severity	*Minor:* Taking into account the reported magnitude of the above-mentioned changes in the metabolism of vitamin B_1 and the large 'therapeutic window' of this substance, the severity of this drug interaction (if any) is probably minor.
Mechanism of action	*No mechanism:* There appears to be no drug interaction between oral contraceptives and vitamin B_1.
Management	No evidence has been obtained indicating that clinically significant effects occur that would require adjustment of the dose or prescription of an alternative medication.
Clinically significant	No.
References	Ahmed F, Bamji MS, Iyengar L. Effect of oral contraceptive agents on vitamin nutrition status. *Am J Clin Nutr* 1975;28:606–15
	Joshi UM, Virkar KD, Amatayakul K, Singkamani R, Bamji MS, Prema K, *et al*. Impact of hormonal contraceptives vis-a-vis non-hormonal factors on the vitamin status of malnourished women in India and Thailand. *Hum Nutr Clin Nutr* 1986;40C: 205–20

References

Lewis CM, King JC. Effect of oral contraceptive agents on thiamine, riboflavin, and pantothenic acid status in young women. *Am J Clin Nutr* 1980;33:832–8

Vir SC, Love AHG. Effect of oral contraceptive agents on thiamine status. *Int J Vitam Nutr Res* 1979;49:292–5

3.18.3 VITAMIN B₂ (RIBOFLAVIN)

Documentation level	*Doubtful:* With regard to vitamin B_2 status, no clinically significant differences between oral contraceptive users and controls have been reported. However, occasional statistically significant decreases in vitamin B_2 plasma concentrations have been observed in oral contraceptive users, but the picture is rather confusing: there seem to be differences in well- and under-nourished oral contraceptive users, as well as between vitamin-supplemented and non-supplemented oral contraceptive users (Sanpitak and Chayutimonkul, 1974; Prasad *et al.*, 1975; Guggenheim and Segal, 1977; Kramer *et al.*, 1977; Vir and Love, 1979; Roe *et al.*, 1982; Tovar *et al.*, 1985; Joshi *et al.*, 1986; Mooij *et al.*, 1991). Analysis of the performed studies by Roe *et al.* (1982) indicated that confounding factors, such as different oral contraceptive formulations, study design, ethnicity, and especially dietary vitamin B_2 intake of the populations studied, may have contributed to the controversy.
Severity	*Minor:* Taking into account the reported magnitude of the above-mentioned changes in the metabolism of vitamin B_2 and the large 'therapeutic window' of this substance, the severity of this drug interaction (if any) is probably minor.
Mechanism of action	*Enzyme induction:* Although a socioeconomic factor cannot be excluded, the different outcome of studies investigating the effect of oral contraceptive use on vitamin B_2 status may be attributed to other external factors, especially to the differences in dietary vitamin B_2 intake between the study populations. An alternative explanation for the above-mentioned suggested deterioration of vitamin B_2 status by oral contraceptive use was given by Capel *et al.* (1981). They found an increased activity of the enzyme erythrocyte glutathione peroxidase in oral contraceptive users as compared to controls. This enzyme counteracts the action of glutathione reductase, which is of crucial importance in determining the vitamin B_2 status. Consequently, this induction of glutathione peroxidase activity may diminish seriously the validity of the test model for assessment of the vitamin B_2 status in humans and, consequently, falsely suggest an effect attributable to oral contraceptive use.
Management	No evidence has been obtained indicating that clinically significant effects occur that would require adjustment of the dose or prescription of an alternative medication.
Clinically significant	No.

References

Capel ID, Jenner M, Williams DC, Donaldson D, Nath A. The effect of prolonged oral contraceptive steroid use on erythrocyte glutathione peroxidase activity. *J Steroid Biochem* 1981;14:729–32

Guggenheim K, Segal S. Oral contraceptives and riboflavin nutriture. *Int J Vitam Nutr Res* 1977;47:234–5

Joshi UM, Virkar KD, Amatayakul K, Singkamani, R, Bamji MS, Prema K, *et al.* Impact of hormonal contraceptives vis-a-vis non-hormonal factors on the vitamin status of malnourished women in India and Thailand. *Hum Nutr Clin Nutr* 1986;40C:205–20

Kramer U, Bitsch R, Hotzel D. Applicability of blood and urine analysis for the determination of nutritional status of riboflavine. *Nutr Metab* 1977;21(Suppl 1):22–3

Mooij PNM, Thomas CMG, Doesburg WH, Eskes TKAB. Multivitamin supplementation in oral contraceptive users. *Contraception* 1991;44:277–88

Prasad AS, Lei KY, Oberleas D, Moghissi KS, Stryker JC. Effect of oral contraceptive agents on nutrients: II Vitamins. *Am J Clin Nutr* 1975;28:385–91

Roe DA, Bogusz S, Sheu J, McCormick DB. Factors affecting riboflavin requirements of oral contraceptive users and non-users. *Am J Clin Nutr* 1982;35:495–501

Sanpitak N, Chayutimonkul L. Oral contraceptives and riboflavin nutrition. *Lancet* 1974;1:836–7

Tovar A, Bourges H, Canto T, Torres N, Lopez-Castro BR. Effect of oral contraceptive use on the erythrocyte glutathione reductase and aspartate aminotransferase activities in women with and without clinical signs of vitamin deficiency. *Nutr Rep Int* 1985;32:199–209

Vir SC, Love AHG. Riboflavin nutriture of oral contraceptive users. *Int J Vitam Nutr Res* 1979;49:286–90

3.18.4 VITAMIN B$_6$ (PYRIDOXINE)

Documentation level

Doubtful: The majority of the early studies suggested that oral contraceptive use altered tryptophan metabolism. The observed changes were similar to those seen in vitamin B$_6$ deficiency and, since they could be corrected by administration of vitamin B$_6$, they have subsequently been interpreted as meaning that oral contraceptive use may lead to vitamin B$_6$ deficiency. However, this tryptophan test model is now considered obsolete, and more appropriate test models do not show significant differences between oral contraceptive users and controls (Leklem, 1986; Bender, 1987). Since both oral contraceptive use and vitamin B$_6$ deficiency have been implicated in the etiology of depression, it has been thought that oral contraceptive-associated depression was due to vitamin B$_6$ depletion.

However, taken together, the available evidence does not support a clinically significant deterioration of vitamin B$_6$ status resulting from oral contraceptive use. Consequently, in the event of a relationship between oral contraceptive use and the occurrence of depressive symptoms, there must be some mechanism other than vitamin B$_6$ depletion that is responsible.

Severity

Minor: Taking into account the reported magnitude of the above-mentioned changes in the metabolism of vitamin B$_6$ and the large 'therapeutic window' of this substance, the severity of this drug interaction (if any) is probably minor.

Mechanism of action

Enzyme inhibition: It has been reported that oral contraceptive use inhibits tryptophan metabolism. However, the tryptophan test model is currently considered obsolete, because estrogens themselves have direct effects (independent from vitamin B$_6$ status) on particular steps of the tryptophan metabolic pathway (via kynureninase inhibition) (Bender *et al.*, 1982; Bender, 1983;1987). Alternative test models, such as measurement of pyridoxal-5'-phosphate and the activation of erythrocyte glutamate oxaloacetate transaminase (a long-term indicator of vitamin B$_6$ status), are now considered as appropriate methods for the assessment of vitamin B$_6$ status (Bior and Bender, 1986; Leklem, 1986). Results of most controlled studies do not show major differences in these parameters between oral contraceptive users and controls (Leklem *et al.*, 1975; Wien, 1978; Bosse and Donald, 1979; Vir and Love, 1980; van der Vange *et al.*, 1989).

Management	No evidence has been obtained indicating that clinically significant effects occur that would require adjustment of the dose or prescription of an alternative medication.
Clinically significant	No.

References

Bender DA, Tagoe CE, Vale JA. Effects of estrogen administration on vitamin B_6 and tryptophan metabolism in the rat. *Br J Nutr* 1982;47:609–14

Bender DA. Effects of estradiol and vitamin B_6 on tryptophan metabolism in the rat: implications for the interpretation of the tryptophan load test for vitamin B_6 nutritional status. *Br J Nutr* 1983;50:33–42

Bender DA. Estrogens and vitamin B_6–actions and interactions. In: *World Review of Nutrition and Diet,* vol. 51. Basel: Karger, 1987:140–88

Bior AD, Bender DA. Aspartate aminotransferase activation by pyridoxal phosphate as an index of vitamin B_6 nutritional status: validity in the presence of estrogen conjugates. *Proc Nutr Soc* 1986;45:59A

Bosse TR, Donald EA. The vitamin B_6 requirement in oral contraceptive users. I. Assessment by pyridoxal level and transferase activity in erythrocytes. *Am J Clin Nutr* 1979;32:1015–23

Leklem JE, Brown RR, Rose DP, Linkswiler H, Ahrend RA. Metabolism of tryptophan and niacin in oral contraceptive users receiving controlled intakes of vitamin B_6. *Am J Clin Nutr* 1975;28:146–56

Leklem JE. Vitamin B_6 requirement and oral contraceptive use–a concern? *J Nutr* 1986;116:475–7

Vange N van der, Berg H van den, Kloosterboer HG, Haspels AA. Effects of seven low-dose combined contraceptives on vitamin B_6 status. *Contraception* 1989;40:377–84

Vir SC, Love AHG. Effect of oral contraceptives on vitamin B_6 nutriture of young women. *Int J Vitam Nutr Res* 1980;50:29–34

Wien EM. Vitamin B_6 status of Nigerian women using various methods of contraception. *Am J Clin Nutr* 1978;31:1392–6

3.18.5 VITAMIN B$_{12}$ (CYANOCOBALAMIN)

Documentation level	*Doubtful:* With regard to vitamin B$_{12}$ status, no clinically significant differences between oral contraceptive users and controls have been reported. However, in general, there is agreement that the use of combined oral contraceptives is associated with decreased serum vitamin B$_{12}$ concentrations (Shojania, 1982; Mountifield, 1985). In addition, the relatively low vitamin B$_{12}$ serum concentrations in oral contraceptive users poorly respond to vitamin B$_{12}$ supplements, suggesting that the lower vitamin B$_{12}$ concentrations in oral contraceptive users do not reflect higher vitamin B$_{12}$ demand (Mountifield, 1986; Mooij *et al.*, 1991). The observed decreased plasma vitamin B$_{12}$ concentrations are not considered of clinical importance, since in the target tissue for vitamin B$_{12}$ (i.e. bone marrow), no decreased concentrations of vitamin B$_{12}$ have been found in oral contraceptive users as compared to controls (Wertalik *et al.*, 1972; Shojania *et al.*, 1979).
Severity	*Minor:* Taking into account the reported magnitude of the above-mentioned changes in the metabolism of vitamin B$_{12}$ and the large 'therapeutic window' of this substance, the severity of this drug interaction (if any) is probably minor.
Mechanism of action	*Protein binding:* The decrease in serum vitamin B$_{12}$ concentration may be due to an oral contraceptive-induced increase in the plasma concentration of the carrier protein for vitamin B$_{12}$, transcobalamin I (Shojania and Wylie, 1979), resulting in an increased binding and possibly also lower free plasma concentrations of vitamin B$_{12}$. From two pivotal studies, it appeared that the observed decrease of vitamin B$_{12}$ serum levels was not related to oral contraceptive dose or type (Shojania and Wylie, 1979; Hjelt *et al.*, 1985). Finally, clinical studies have shown that vitamin B$_{12}$ absorption and urinary excretion are not impaired in oral contraceptive users (Shojania and Wylie, 1979; Hjelt *et al.*, 1985).
Management	No evidence has been obtained indicating that clinically significant effects occur that would require adjustment of the dose or prescription of an alternative medication.
Clinically significant	No.

References

Hjelt K, Brynskov J, Hippe E, Lundstrom P, Munck O. Oral contraceptives and the cobalamin (vitamin B_{12}) metabolism. *Acta Obstet Gynecol Scand* 1985;64:59–63

Mooij PNM, Thomas CMG, Doesburg WH, Eskes TKAB. Multivitamin supplementation in oral contraceptive users. *Contraception* 1991;44:277–88

Mountifield JA. Effects of oral contraceptive usage on B_{12} and folate levels. *Can Fam Phys* 1985;31:1523–6

Mountifield JA. Serum vitamin B_{12} and folate levels in women taking oral contraceptives. *Can Fam Phys* 1986;32:862–5

Shojania AM, Wylie B. The effect of oral contraceptives on vitamin B_{12} metabolism. *Am J Obstet Gynecol* 1979;135:129–34

Shojania AM. Oral contraceptives: effects on folate and vitamin B_{12} metabolism. *Can Med Assoc J* 1982;126:244–7

Wertalik LF, Metz EN, LoBuglio AF, Balcerzak SP. Decreased serum B_{12} levels with oral contraceptive use. *J Am Med Assoc* 1972;221:1371–4

3.18.6 VITAMIN C

3.18.6a Effect of oral contraceptives on vitamin C pharmacokinetics

Documentation level	*Doubtful:* According to the early literature, the use of combined oral contraceptives by women is associated with decreased concentrations of vitamin C (ascorbic acid) in plasma (Rivers and Devine, 1972; Harris *et al.*, 1975), in platelets (Kalesh *et al.*, 1971), and in leukocytes (McLeroy and Schendel, 1973) as compared to controls. However, in none of these studies (in which the former higher dose oral contraceptive regimens had been used) were the ascorbic acid plasma concentrations found to be below the normal range of 0.40–0.60 mg/dl (Hudiburgh and Milner, 1979). More recent studies have indicated that plasma vitamin C concentrations in oral contraceptive users are not decreased in comparison to controls (Horwitt *et al.*, 1975; Yeung, 1976; Hudiburgh and Milner, 1979; Cummings, 1981; Basu *et al.*, 1989; Mooij *et al.*, 1991).
Severity	*Minor:* Taking into account the reported magnitude of the above-mentioned changes in the metabolism of vitamin C and the large 'therapeutic window' of this substance, the severity of this drug interaction (if any) is probably minor.
Mechanism of action	*Unknown:* The available information is contradictory and controversy exists about the mechanism of action. Suggestions include increased catabolism, decreased absorption, changes in tissue distribution, and decreased levels of reducing compounds such as reduced glutathione (Rivers, 1975).
Management	No evidence has been obtained indicating that clinically significant effects occur that would require adjustment of the dose or prescription of an alternative medication.
Clinically significant	No.

3.18.6b Effect of vitamin C on oral contraceptive pharmacokinetics

Documentation level	*Possible:* In pharmacokinetic interaction studies in female hamsters (Rovagnati *et al.*, 1982) and in women (Back *et al.*, 1981), it appeared that the concurrent use of combined oral contraceptives and vitamin C (ascorbic acid) resulted in increased plasma concentrations of ethinylestradiol as compared to plasma ethinylestradiol levels before ascorbic acid supplementation.

Severity	*Minor:* Taking into account the absence of ethinylestradiol-related side-effects in women using oral contraceptives and ascorbic acid concurrently, and the large inter- and intraindividual variations in ethinylestradiol plasma levels, the severity of this interaction is probably minor.
Mechanism of action	*Absorption:* The increased bioavailability of ethinylestradiol can probably be attributed to a competitively (versus ascorbic acid) impaired sulfate conjugation of ethinylestradiol in the intestinal mucosa, resulting in a reduced first-pass effect and thus an increased intestinal absorption. In addition, the increased plasma concentrations of ethinylestradiol after concurrent use of ascorbic acid are also evidenced by increased plasma levels of some ethinylestradiol-sensitive plasma proteins (Back *et al.*, 1981).
Management	No evidence has been obtained indicating that clinically significant effects occur that would require adjustment of the dose or prescription of an alternative medication.
Clinically significant	No.

References	Back DJ, Breckenridge AM, MacIver M, Orme ML'E, Purba H, Rowe PH. Interaction of ethinylestradiol with ascorbic acid in man. *Br Med J* 1981;282:1516–17
	Basu J, Vermund SH, Mikhail M, Palan PR, Romney SL. Plasma reduced and total ascorbic acid in healthy women: effects of smoking and oral contraception. *Contraception* 1989;39:85–93
	Cummings FJ. Effect of oral contraceptive use on ascorbic acid and vitamin A in lactation. *J Hum Nutr* 1981;35:249–56
	Harris AB, Pillay M, Hussein S. Vitamins and oral contraceptives. *Lancet* 1975;2:82–3
	Horwitt MK, Harvey CC, Dahm CH. Relationship between levels of blood lipids, vitamins C, A and E, serum copper compounds, and urinary excretions of tryptophan metabolites in women taking oral contraceptive therapy. *Am J Clin Nutr* 1975;28:403–12
	Hudiburgh NK, Milner AN. Influences of oral contraceptives on ascorbic acid and triglyceride status. *J Am Diet Assoc* 1979:75:19–22

References

Kalesh DG, Mallikarjuneswara VR, Clemetson CAB. Effect of estrogen-containing oral contraceptives on platelet and plasma ascorbic acid concentrations. *Contraception* 1971;4:183–92

McLeroy J, Schendel HE. Influence of oral contraceptives on ascorbic acid concentrations in healthy, sexually mature women. *Am J Clin Nutr* 1973;26:191–6

Mooij PNM, Thomas CMG, Doesburg WH, Eskes TKAB. Multivitamin supplementation in oral contraceptive users. *Contraception* 1991;44:277–88

Rivers JM, Devine MM. Plasma ascorbic acid concentrations and oral contraceptives. *Am J Clin Nutr* 1972;25:684–9

Rivers JM. Oral contraceptives and ascorbic acid. *Am J Clin Nutr* 1975;28:550–4

Rovagnati P, Di Padova C, Di Padova F, Munari L, Tritapepe R. Effect of a concomitant treatment with ethinylestradiol and ascorbic acid on bile secretion in female hamsters. *Meth Find Exp Clin Pharmacol* 1982;4:313–16

Yeung DL. Relationship between cigarette smoking, oral contraceptives and plasma vitamins A, E, C, and plasma triglycerides and cholesterol. *Am J Clin Nutr* 1976;29:1216–21

3.18.7 VITAMIN D

Documentation level	*Doubtful:* Several studies have suggested that the pharmaco-kinetics of vitamin D in oral contraceptive users may be different from that in non-users. Carter *et al.* (1975) found an increased elimination half-life of vitamin D_3 in oral contraceptive users as compared to controls. Other studies showed that oral contraceptive users had slightly higher plasma concentrations of bound plus unbound calcitriol, but not of total vitamin D_2. The free plasma concentrations of both vitamin D_3 and calcitriol remained unaffected (Bouillon *et al.*, 1977;1981). In addition, a long-term study by Schreurs *et al.* (1981) also did not show any differences between oral contraceptive users and controls with respect to total plasma vitamin D_2 concentrations. Finally, Gray *et al.* (1982) showed that oral contraceptive users did not manifest a mid-cycle peak of plasma calcitriol (in contrast to non-users), indicating an influence of ovarian function and endogenous estrogens on the metabolism of calcitriol.
Severity	*Minor:* Taking into account the reported magnitude of the above-mentioned changes in the metabolism of vitamin D and the large 'therapeutic window' of this substance, the severity of this drug interaction (if any) is probably minor.
Mechanism of action	*Protein binding:* The increase in the plasma concentration of total calcitriol in oral contraceptive users was attributed to an estrogen-induced increase in the hepatic synthesis of vitamin D-binding protein, similar to the increase of other estrogen-sensitive plasma proteins during oral contraceptive use (Haddad and Walgate, 1976; Haddad *et al.*, 1976; Bouillon *et al.*, 1981).
Management	No evidence has been obtained indicating that clinically significant effects occur that would require adjustment of the dose or prescription of an alternative medication.
Clinically significant	No.

References	Bouillon R, Baelen H van, Moor P de. The measurement of the vitamin D-binding protein in human serum. *J Clin Endocrinol Metab* 1977;45:225–31

References

Bouillon R, Assche FA van, Baelen H van, Heyns W, Moor P de. Influence of the vitamin D-binding protein on the serum concentration of 1,25-dihydroxyvitamin D₃. *J Clin Invest* 1981;67:589–96

Carter DE, Bressler R, Hughes MR, Haussler MR, Christian CD, Heine MW. Effect of oral contraceptives on plasma clearance. *Clin Pharmacol Ther* 1975;18:700–7

Gray TK, McAdoo T, Hatley L, Lester GE, Thierry M. Fluctuation of serum concentration of 1,25–dihydroxyvitamin D₃ during the menstrual cycle. *Am J Obstet Gynecol* 1982;144:880–4

Haddad JG, Walgate J. Radioimmunoassay of the binding protein for vitamin D and its metabolites in human serum. *J Clin Invest* 1976;58:1217–22

Haddad JG, Hillman L, Rojanasathit S. Human serum binding capacity and affinity for 25-hydroxyergocalciferol and 25-hydroxycalciferol. *J Clin Endocrinol Metab* 1976;43:86–91

Schreurs WHP, Rijn HJM van, Berg H van den. Serum 25-hydroxycholecalciferol levels in women using oral contraceptives. *Contraception* 1981;23:399–406

3.18.8 VITAMIN E

Documentation level	*Doubtful:* Early studies in rats (Aftergood and Alfin-Slater, 1973; Aftergood *et al.*, 1976) and some studies in women showed decreased plasma concentrations of α-tocopherol during the administration of contraceptive steroids as compared to controls (Aftergood *et al.*, 1975; Martino *et al.*, 1988). Other studies failed to show an effect of oral contraceptive use on plasma α-tocopherol levels (Horwitt *et al.*, 1975; Yeung, 1976; Jagadeesan and Prema, 1980). One study even showed increased plasma α-tocopherol levels associated with oral contraceptive use (Smith *et al.*, 1975). In addition, in a controlled study Tangney and Driskell (1978) reported that plasma α-tocopherol was reduced in oral contraceptive users who took daily norethisterone/mestranol at a dose of 1000/80 µg/day, whereas there was no change in users of norethisterone/mestranol at a dose of 1000/50 µg/day, which suggested an estrogen dose-dependency. The latter suggestion is supported by the finding that low-dose progestagen-only preparations had no effect on plasma α-tocopherol concentrations (Yeung and Chan, 1975). However, clinically relevant interactions have not been reported.
Severity	*Minor:* Taking into account the reported magnitude of the above-mentioned changes in the metabolism of vitamin E and the large 'therapeutic window' of this substance, the severity of this drug interaction (if any) is probably minor.
Mechanism of action	*Protein binding:* The suggested mechanism of action for the variability in plasma α-tocopherol levels in oral contraceptive users is an effect on plasma lipoproteins, because these lipoproteins are also capable of binding α-tocopherol. Oral contraceptives could, therefore, depending on their estrogen content, exert some influence on the binding of α-tocopherol to plasma lipoproteins (Smith *et al.*, 1975; Yeung and Chan, 1975; Jagadeesan and Prema, 1980). Recently, it was shown that a decrease in plasma α-tocopherol levels was associated with a decrease of the plasma low-density lipoprotein (LDL) fraction (Martino *et al.*, 1988), suggesting that LDL is the carrier for α-tocopherol in plasma.
Management	No evidence has been obtained indicating that clinically significant effects occur that would require adjustment of the dose or prescription of an alternative medication.
Clinically significant	No.

References

Aftergood L, Alfin-Slater RB. Oral contraceptive–α-tocopherol interrelationships. *Lipids* 1973;9:91–6

Aftergood L, Alexander AR, Alfin-Slater RB. Effect of oral contraceptives on plasma lipoproteins, cholesterol and α-tocopherol levels in young women. *Nutr Rep Int* 1975;11:295–304

Aftergood L, Fields JE, Alfin-Slater RB. Effect of an oral contraceptive on α-tocopherol levels in rat tissues. *Nutr Rep Int* 1976;13:217–24

Horwitt MK, Harvey CC, Dahm CH. Relationship between levels of blood lipids, vitamins C, A and E, serum copper compounds, and urinary excretions of tryptophan metabolites in women taking oral contraceptive therapy. *Am J Clin Nutr* 1975;28:403–12

Jagadeesan V, Prema K. Plasma tocopherol and lipid levels in pregnancy and oral contraceptive users. *Br J Obstet Gynaecol* 1980;87:903–7

Martino F, Lapiana C, Di Salvo G, Galati G, Avitto P, Lubrano R. Effetti della somministrazione orale di un contraccettivo sull'assetto lipidico e sulla concentrazione di tocoferolo sierico. *Min Ginecol* 1988;40:557–8

Smith JL, Goldsmith GA, Lawrence JD. Effects of oral contraceptive steroids on vitamin and lipid levels in serum. *Am J Clin Nutr* 1975;28:371–6

Tangney CC, Driskell JA. Vitamin E status of young women on combined-type oral contraceptives. *Contraception* 1978;17:499–512

Yeung DL, Chan PL. Effect of a progestogen and a sequential type oral contraceptive on plasma vitamin A, vitamin E, cholesterol and triglycerides. *Am J Clin Nutr* 1975;28:686–91

Yeung DL. Relationship between cigarette smoking, oral contraceptives, and plasma vitamins A, E, C, and plasma triglycerides and cholesterol. *Am J Clin Nutr* 1976;29:1216–21

3.18.9 FOLIC ACID

Documentation level	*Doubtful:* Early reports suggested an association of the use of oral contraceptives with both decreased plasma and erythrocyte folic acid concentrations (Shojania *et al.*, 1971;1975; Smith *et al.*, 1975; Hettiarachchy *et al.*, 1983). However, many other studies have failed to substantiate these findings (Pritchard *et al.*, 1971; Stephens *et al.*, 1972; Butterworth *et al.*, 1975; Paine *et al.*, 1975; Ross *et al.*, 1976; Mountifield, 1986; Mooij *et al.*, 1991). Some authors have attributed cases of megaloblastic anemia, accidentally observed in oral contraceptive users, to these decreased folic acid plasma levels (Whitehead *et al.*, 1973; Meguid and Loebi, 1974). Most studies, however, show increased values of hematological parameters in oral contraceptive users as compared to non-users, even after correction for decreased menstrual blood loss (Shojania *et al.*, 1982). From these data, it is concluded that, with the former higher dose oral contraceptive regimens, some deterioration of folate status cannot be excluded. However, this effect is probably mild and unlikely to cause megaloblastic anemia in healthy oral contraceptive users. In studies using modern low-dose oral contraceptives, no effects on plasma folic acid levels have been observed.
Severity	*Minor:* Taking into account the reported magnitude of the above-mentioned changes in the metabolism of folic acid and the large 'therapeutic window' of this substance, the severity of this drug interaction (if any) is probably minor.
Mechanism of action	*Excretion:* The decreased folic acid plasma concentrations reported in users of higher dose oral contraceptive regimens have been attributed to an increased urinary excretion of folic acid intermediates (Gaafar *et al.*, 1973; Shojania *et al.*, 1975). Other proposed mechanisms are increased folic acid metabolism due to enzyme induction (Maxwell *et al.*, 1972) and increased plasma protein binding of folic acid (Da Costa and Rothenberg, 1974). The increased folic acid excretion in oral contraceptive users could not be confirmed by Butterworth *et al.* (1975); neither have the other proposed mechanisms of action been confirmed.
Management	No evidence has been obtained indicating that clinically significant effects occur that would require adjustment of the dose or prescription of an alternative medication.
Clinically significant	No.

References

Butterworth CE, Krumdieck CL, Stinson HN, Cornwell PE. A study of the effect of oral contraceptive agents on the absorption, metabolic conversion and urinary excretion of a naturally-occurring folate (citrovorum factor). *Ala J Med Sci* 1975;12:330–5

Da Costa M, Rothenberg SP. Appearance of a folate binder in leukocytes and serum of women who are pregnant or taking oral contraceptives. *J Lab Clin Med* 1974;83:207–14

Gaafar A, Toppozada HK, Hozayen A, Abdel-Malek AT, Moghazy M, Youssef M. Study of folate status in long-term Egyptian users of oral contraceptive pills. *Contraception* 1973;8:43–52

Hettiarachchy NS, Sri Kantha SS, Corea SMX. The effect of oral contraceptive therapy and of pregnancy on serum folate levels of rural Sri Lankan women. *Br J Nutr* 1983;50:495–501

Maxwell JD, Hunter J, Steward DA, Ardeman S, Williams R. Folate deficiency after anticonvulsant drugs: an effect of hepatic enzyme induction? *Br Med J* 1972;1:297–9

Meguid MM, Loebi WY. Megaloblastic anemia associated with the oral contraceptive pill. *Postgrad Med J* 1974;50:470–2

Mooij PNM, Thomas CMG, Doesburg WH, Eskes TKAB. Multivitamin supplementation in oral contraceptive users. *Contraception* 1991;44:277–88

Mountifield JA. Serum vitamin B_{12} and folate levels in women taking oral contraceptives. *Can Fam Phys* 1986;32:862–5

Paine CJ, Grafton WD, Dickson VL, Eichner ER. Oral contraceptives, serum folate, and hematologic status. *J Am Med Assoc* 1975;231:731–3

Pritchard JA, Scott DE, Whalley PJ. Maternal folate deficiency and pregnancy wastage. IV. Effects of folic acid supplements, anticonvulsants, and oral contraceptives. *Am J Obstet Gynecol* 1971;109:341–6

Ross CE, Stone MK, Reagan JW, Wentz WB, Kellermeyer RW. Lack of influence of oral contraceptives on serum folate, hematologic values, and uterine cervical cytology. *Semin Hematol* 1976;13:233–8

References

Shojania AM, Hornady GJ, Barnes PH. The effect of oral contraceptives on folate metabolism. *Am J Obstet Gynecol* 1971;111:782–91

Shojania AM, Hornady GJ, Scaletta D. The effect of oral contraceptives on folate metabolism. III. Plasma clearance and urinary folate excretion. *J Lab Clin Med* 1975;85:185–90

Shojania AM. Oral contraceptives: effects on folate and vitamin B_{12} metabolism. *Can Med Assoc J* 1982;126:244–7

Smith JL, Goldsmith GA, Lawrence JD. Effects of oral contraceptive steroids on vitamin and lipid levels in serum. *Am J Clin Nutr* 1975;28:371–6

Stephens MEM, Craft I, Peters TJ, Hoffbrand AV. Oral contraceptives and folate metabolism. *Clin Sci* 1972;42:405–14

Whitehead N, Reyner F, Lindenbaum J. Megaloblastic changes in the cervical epithelium. *J Am Med Assoc* 1973;226:1421–4

Index